The Fight Against HIV Continues: High Prevalence Persists Despite Progress

Nicholas

First Printing, 2024

TABLE OF CONTENTS

CHAPTER 1 :LITERATURE REVIEW

1.1 Introduction

The World Health Organization (WHO) reported that an estimated 37.9 million people were HIV infected in 2018 worldwide, with an estimated global prevalence of 0.8% (UNAIDS, 2018; **Figure 1**). Sub-Saharan Africa carries the heaviest burden of HIV infections with 68% of infections found in this region, (Ledergerber & Battegay, 2014). In South Africa (SA), about 7.1 million people were reported to be HIV-infected by 2016. Of these, 4.1 million (57.7%) were women, while 320,000 were children between 0-14 years old. The prevalence of HIV in SA adults of reproductive age (15-49 years) was 20.4% in 2018 (UNAIDS, 2018).

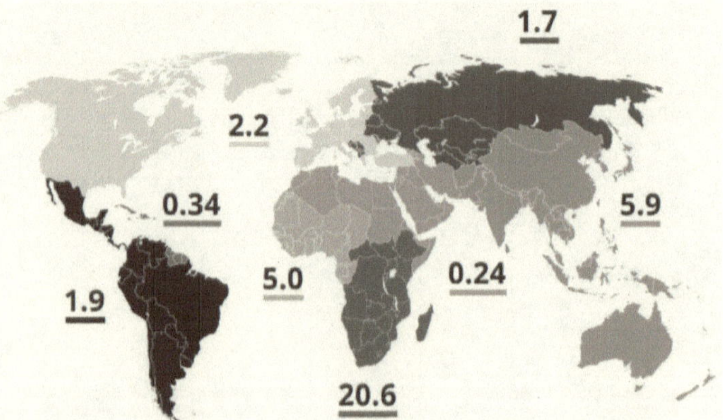

Figure 1.1: Worldwide distribution of HIV infections in 2018 (source: UNAIDS, 2018).

1.2 HIV infection

1.2.1 Transmission of HIV

The transmission of HIV from one individual to another can occur across mucosal surfaces through unprotected sexual intercourse, exchange of body fluids, sharing of needles in injection drug use or vertically through mother-to-child transmission (Correa & Gisselquist, 2006). Heterosexual transmission is the most common mode of transmission accounting for approximately 86% of all

HIV infections (Simon *et al.*, 2006). Injection drug use and transmission between male partners account for a considerable proportion of the remainder of infections (Kalichman *et al.*, 2006). Comparing the two genders, transmission rates are said to be greater from males to females than vice versa, highlighting the importance of having a better understanding of the FGT and HIV acquisition in women (Gosmann *et al.*, 2017).

The risk of sexual HIV transmission from an infected individual to an uninfected partner correlates positively with partner HIV viral load (Quinn *et al.*, 2000; Marks *et al.*, 2016). Additionally, there is a wide range of other biological and behavioural risk factors, including sexually transmitted infections (STIs), non-circumcision in men, immunological status of infected individuals, the frequency of sexual contact, gender-based violence, transmission networks and intergenerational sex, pregnancy, cervical ectopy and lack of antiretroviral therapy in infected individuals (Quinn *et al.*, 2000; de Oliviera *et al.*, 2017). Recent studies have shown that elevated concentrations of chemokines and proinflammatory cytokines in the FGT prior to sexual contact markedly increases the risk of HIV acquisition (Masson *et al.*, 2015; McKinnon *et al.*, 2018). Additionally, women with non-optimal bacterial communities in their FGTs, who have high levels of inflammatory cytokines, are at greater risk of HIV acquisition compared to women with *Lactobacillus*-dominated microbiota (Eastment *et al.*, 2015; Gosmann *et al.*, 2017; Lennard *et al.*, 2017). Therefore, understanding the biological factors in the FGT that influence HIV acquisition risk is critical for the development of strategies to prevent HIV infection in women.

1.3 Defense mechanisms of the FGT

1.3.1 Adaptive immune responses in the FGT

Adaptive immune responses are made up of two types of lymphocytes, B (humoral) and T cells (cell-mediated), which express a large repertoire of antigen-specific receptors known as B-cell and T-cell receptors (Vivier *et al.*, 2011). Naïve B and T-cells come into contact with antigens in lymphoid organs and this triggers a cell division and maturation process before initiation of effector functions (Vivier *et al.*, 2011). For an effective immune response to be mounted against pathogens, antigen presenting cells (APCs) are required to process the antigen before presenting it to T-cells and therefore activating the T-cells during a cell-mediated immune response. APCs include macrophages, DCs, Langerhans cells and also epithelial cells (Hickey et al., 2011). On the other hand, the humoral immune response is mediated by antibodies that are produced by B-cells. Macrophages phagocytose pathogens and present the antigens to T-helper cells. Thereafter, T-helper cells bind to the macrophage and become activated. The activated T-helper cells then bind to B-cells in order to activate the B-cells (Abbas *et al.*, 2016). After antigen presentation, a cascade of processes is activated, including antibody synthesis, and cytokine production.

The production of inflammatory cytokines plays a major role in fighting sexually transmitted and viral pathogens (Svanborg *et al.*, 1999; Wira *et al.*, 2005). Cytokines are pleiotropic proteins with the critical role of mediating communication between the immune system and host tissue cells (Amjadi *et al.*, 2014; Mcinnes *et al.*, 2017). The cytokines produced in response to pathogens determine whether the type of response is humoral, cytotoxic or cell mediated (Borish & Steinke, 2003).

1.3.2 Innate immunity in the vaginal mucosa

1.3.2.1 Mechanical barriers

Immunity in the lower FGT can be grouped into innate and adaptive immune systems (Wira *et al.*, 2005), both of which are critical protective mechanisms against pathogens in the FGT (Mirmonsef *et al.*, 2011). The two responses differ in the specificity of receptors, the timing of response, immune cells involved and the effector mechanisms employed (Amjadi *et al.*, 2014). The innate immune system consists of mechanical, chemical and cellular components (Amjadi *et al.*, 2014). The first line of innate immune defense against pathogens in the lower FGT is the mucosal mechanical barrier which is composed of non-keratinised stratified squamous epithelium and a layer of mucus. The upper genital tract is covered by a single layer of columnar epithelium (Nasioudis *et al.*, 2017; Petrova *et al.*, 2013; Wira *et al.*, 2005) which is more vulnerable to HIV transmission, although the presence of a thick mucus layer and tight junctions between cells provide a barrier that efficiently traps HIV virions (Hladik & Hope, 2019). The vaginal epithelium has distinct features such as basal cells which act as progenitors for the apical layers (Rose *et al.*, 2012). The epithelium forms a protective barrier that separates the interior of the body and the outside environment. This innate immune barrier prevents the dissemination of pathogens such as bacteria, viruses, parasites and fungi due to the presence of tight junctions and secretion of mucus which covers the vaginal and cervical surfaces and traps infectious organisms (Mirmonsef *et al.*, 2011). In addition to trapping and excluding microorganisms, the mucus acts as a medium for a number of antimicrobial peptides and proteins such as defensins (Valore *et al.*, 2002). Permeability of the tight junctions varies to allow innate immune cells to pass through (Rose *et al.*, 2012). The mucosal epithelium in the vagina is constantly colonised by microorganisms, making it a non-sterile environment (Petrova *et al.*, 2013). Additionally, the lower FGT is well adapted to be tolerant of hormonal cycling throughout a woman's reproductive life and also various exogenous stimuli introduced during sexual intercourse (Kunz *et al.*, 1997).

1.3.2.2 Chemical and cellular barriers

The chemical and cellular components of the innate immune response are non-specific and activated when the immune and non-immune cells encounter pathogens (Luster, 2002). Innate immune responses are rapid, non-specific and rely on recognition of conserved molecules expressed by pathogens (Quayle *et al.*, 2002). These early responses help to prevent the establishment of infections until antigen-specific cells have been recruited to the site (Quayle, 2002). The chemical barrier comprises antimicrobial peptides (AMPs) and cytokines while the cellular component involves pattern recognition receptors (PRRs) such as toll-like receptors (TLR) (Nasu *et al.*, 2010; Hickey *et al.*, 2011). PRRs are expressed on the surface of neutrophils, macrophages, dendritic cells (DCs), dermal endothelial cells, and mucosal epithelial cells (Fazeli *et al.*, 2005; Wiesner & Vilcinskas, 2010). The recognition of pathogens takes place when PRRs identify and bind to microbe-associated molecular patterns and initiate intracellular signaling pathways to recruit immune cells which in turn secrete antimicrobial factors and cytokines (Medzhitov *et al.*, 1998; Amjadi *et al.*, 2014). Secreted cytokines and chemokines include tumor necrosis factor (TNF)-α, granulocyte-colony stimulating factor (G-CSF), granulocyte-macrophage colony stimulating factor (GM-CSF), interleukin (IL)-6, and IL-8, which recruit immune cells and/or induce cellular activation and differentiation for a successful immune response (Wira *et al.*, 2005; Wira *et al.*, 2010). This results in the disruption of pathogen replication and eradication, although these types of responses are non-specific (Mirmonsef *et al.*, 2011). If the epithelial barrier is compromised, pathogens will encounter a second defense layer consisting of specialized immune cells and cell products (Wira *et al.*, 2005; Wira *et al.*, 2010). The primary immune cells involved include macrophages, DCs, and natural killer (NK) cells, which can take up, process and destroy pathogens (Mirmonsef *et al.*, 2011). The distribution of innate immune cells in the FGT varies depending on site, menstrual cycle and reproductive hormone levels (Wira *et al.*, 2005; Petrova *et al.*, 2013).

1.3.2.3 Optimal vaginal microbiota as a defense mechanism

1.3.2.3.1 Optimal vaginal microbiota

Commensal bacteria are associated with the general health of the vaginal mucosa (Anahtar *et al.*, 2018; Rose *et al.*, 2012). Some of the most common species isolated from the FGT include *Lactobacillus*, *Prevotella*, *Anaerococcus*, *Sneathia*, *Gardnerella*, *Corynebacterium* and *Megasphaera* (McKinnon *et al.*, 2019; Nunn & Forney, 2016). The bacterial composition has been shown to change over time due to changes in estrogen levels during the maturation of a woman (Burton *et al.*, 2003; Heinemann & Reid, 2005; Raz *et al.*, 2003; Brotman, Ravel, Cone, & Zenilman, 2010; Gajer *et al.*, 2012). Maternal estrogen circulating in the infant after birth facilitates the thickening of the vaginal epithelium during the early stages of infancy and regulates deposition of glycogen in epithelial cells. Glycogen is released during exfoliation of the epithelial cells, providing glucose as a source of carbohydrate for lactobacilli in the FGT (Boskey *et al.*, 2001). During early childhood, the vagina is mostly dominated by Gram negative bacteria due to low levels of glycogen present in the vaginal mucosa (Dei *et al.*, 2010; Randelović *et al.*, 2012). At puberty, estrogen facilitates the thickening of the mucosal lining and the glycogen rich environment favors the growth of glucose-fermenting micro-organisms, such as lactobacilli (Mirmonsef *et al.*, 2016). The vaginal microbiota in adolescent girls is similar to adult women (Yamamoto *et al.*, 2009). **Figure 1.2** illustrates the changes in the vaginal mucosa at different stages in a woman's life. Interestingly, it has been shown that bacterial vaginosis (BV)-associated pathogens or non-optimal microbiota such as *G. vaginalis* strains are also capable of catabolizing glycogen in FGT, suggesting competition for nutrients between lactobacilli and anaerobic bacteria in the FGT (Yeoman *et al.*, 2010). The ability of *G. vaginalis* species to catabolise glycogen may also suggest that the changes in microbiota over time are not entirely dependent on glycogen as previously believed (Mirmonsef *et al.*, 2016).

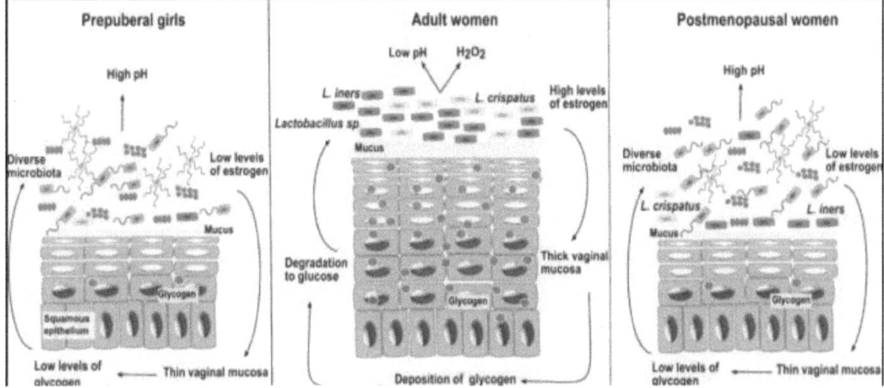

Figure 1.2: The vaginal mucosa during prepuberal, adult and postmenopausal stages of a woman's life. In prepuberal females, the low levels of glycogen present in the vaginal mucosa result in a diverse bacterial community. At puberty and in adult women, the glycogen rich environment promotes the growth of glucose-fermenting micro-organisms such as lactobacilli. In postmenopausal women, the levels of estrogen decline and the environment favors the growth of diverse species. Figure adopted from (Petrova *et al.*, 2013).

An optimal vaginal microbiota is mostly dominated by *Lactobacillus* species (Ravel *et al.*, 2011; Martínez-Peña *et al.*, 2013; Anahtar *et al.*, 2015). Studies have shown that the most common *Lactobacillus* spp. isolated from the genital tracts of healthy pre-menopausal women include *L. iners, L. crispatus, L. gasseri, L. jensenii, L. acidophilus, L. fermentum, L. plantarum, L. brevis, L. casei, L. vaginalis, L. delbrueckii, L. salivarius, L. reuteri,* and *L. rhamnosus* (Anukam *et al.*, 2005; Fredricks *et al.*, 2005; Ravel *et al.*, 2011; Gosmann *et al.*, 2017; McKinnon *et al.*, 2019). The majority of the women with *Lactobacillus* dominated microbiota are Caucasian women of European or American origin (Allsworth & Peipert, 2007; Fettweis *et al.*, 2014; Ravel *et al.*, 2011). A considerable proportion of seemingly healthy asymptomatic African and Hispanic women have a vaginal microbiota that is not dominated by *Lactobacillus* species (Allsworth & Peipert, 2007; Ravel *et al.*, 2011; Fettweis *et al.*, 2014). Although *L. crispatus* has been the most common species associated with health in the FGTs of Caucasian women, it is less frequently isolated from South African women (Anahtar *et al.*, 2015; Klatt *et al.*, 2017; Lennard *et al.*, 2017).

In the past, only culture dependent methods were used to identify bacteria in the FGT, before the development of molecular methods. These methods failed to isolate certain species such as *L. iners,* which can only be grown on blood agar instead of the standard lactobacilli culture medium, de Man Rogosa and Sharpe (MRS) (Sharpe, 1960). The role of *L. iners* in vaginal health is still not well understood since it has been isolated from women considered to have an optimal microbiome, asymptomatic women, as well as women with non-optimal microbiota (Verstraelen *et al.*, 2009). Interestingly, *L. iners* has also been associated with the recovery state in women after antibiotic treatment (Rose *et al.*, 2012). It has been reported that *L. iners* has a very small genome with genes that are responsible for its ability to adapt to fluctuations in the vaginal environment (Macklaim *et al.*, 2011), which may explain how frequently the species is isolated from women with varying microbiota (Burton & Reid, 2002; Srinivasan *et al.*, 2012; Thies *et al.*, 2007; Wertz *et al.*, 2008). Additionally, *L. iners* has also been associated with upregulation of inflammatory cytokine production in vaginal epithelial cells *in vitro* (Doerflinger *et al.*, 2014). Studies have shown that there are several different microbial community types in the FGT, although different studies have identified varying groupings (Witkin *et al.*, 2007; Ravel *et al.*, 2011; Gajer *et al.*, 2012; Anahtar *et al.*, 2015; Lennard *et al.*, 2017; McKinnon *et al.*, 2019). Groupings are determined by unsupervised clustering approaches and are primarily distinguished by the predominant bacterial species. Identification of the predominant species has been shown to be influenced by sample type used, region of the 16S rRNA gene that is amplified and analysis approaches employed, which may account for some of the differences observed from one population to another (McKinnon *et al.*, 2019; Petrova *et al.*, 2017; Ravel *et al.*, 2011). In a recent study by McKinnon *et al.*, fourteen possible groups of vaginal microbiota were identified (McKinnon *et al.*, 2019). Eight of the groups were dominated by *L. crispatus*, *L. jensenii*, *L. gasseri* and *L. iners* while the rest were dominated by anaerobic bacteria such as *Prevotella*, *Sneathia*, *Gardnerella* and *Megasphaera* species.

1.3.2.3.2 Protective mechanisms of optimal vaginal microbiota

As mentioned above, a vaginal microbiota dominated by lactobacilli seems to play a crucial role in the prevention of urogenital infections including HIV (Brotman *et al.*, 2010; Cherpes *et al.*, 2003; Rathod *et al.*, 2012). Young women of African origin who have *L. crispatus*-dominated microbiota were shown to be at a lower risk of HIV acquisition compared with women whose microbiomes were dominated by *L. iners* or diverse anaerobes (Gosmann *et al.*, 2017). Suggested mechanisms of protection include direct inhibition by production of lactic acid, hydrogen peroxide and bacteriocins or indirect mechanisms such as inhibition of the growth of pathogens and regulation of the immune system (Aldunate *et al.*, 2015; Gong *et al.*, 2014; Gosmann *et al.*, 2017; Hearps *et al.*, 2017; Witkin *et al.*, 2015; Arena *et al.*, 2018; El-Adawi *et al.*, 2015; Mastromarino *et al.*, 2011).

Hydrogen peroxide (H_2O_2) produced by lactobacilli has a virucidal effect on HIV, inhibiting viral adhesion and replication (Klebanoff and Coombs., 1991). It has been shown that H_2O_2-producing lactobacilli are present in most of the women with optimal vaginal microbiota compared to those with non-optimal microbiota, suggesting an important protective role played by lactobacilli against BV. A previous study investigated the capacity of a collection of lactobacilli isolates, obtained from healthy Spanish premenopausal women, to produce H_2O_2 and found that *L. jensenii* isolates generated large amounts of H_2O_2 while *L. crispatus* and *L. gasseri* strains produced variable amounts (Martin and Suaírez., 2010). However, it has been shown that lactobacilli do not produce large amounts of H_2O_2 under anaerobic conditions similar to those found in the vagina compared to aerobic conditions (Ocana.,1999). This may suggest that H_2O_2 produced in the vagina may not reach microbicidal concentrations. Additionally, when H_2O_2 was added to *in vitro* cultures at microbicidal concentrations, lactobacilli were inactivated more effectively compared to BV-associated bacteria (Hanlon *et al.*, 2011).

Lactic acid, produced by lactobacilli, maintains a physiological pH below 4.5 in the genital tract (Aroutcheva *et al.*, 2001; Valore *et al.*, 2002; Yeoman *et al.*, 2013). This low pH hinders the growth of potential pathogens, renders HIV virus particles inactive, and may also prevent activation of HIV target cells (Aldunate *et al.*, 2013; Tyssen *et al.*, 2018). The low pH may also aid in lysing exfoliated vaginal epithelial cells which then release glycogen into the vaginal lumen to be utilised by lactobacilli (Nasioudis *et al.*, 2017). In women with non-optimal microbiota, there is a marked depletion in lactic acid in the lower FGT (Aldunate *et al.*, 2015; Hearps *et al.*, 2017), resulting in an increase in vaginal pH. Lactic acid exists as L- and D- isomers, most of which are produced by lactobacilli (Tachedjian *et al.*, 2017). L-lactic acid has been reported to be more effective at inactivating HIV than D-lactate (Aldunate *et al.*, 2015), while D-lactate is mostly active against bacterial STIs such as *Chlamydia trachomatis* (Gong *et al.*, 2014; Nardini *et al.*, 2016). Bacteriocins produced by lactobacilli have bactericidal effects by permeabilizing the membranes of pathogenic Gram-negative bacteria (Danielsson *et al*., 2011). Studies have also investigated the use of bacteriocins as antiviral agents and showed inhibition against HSV-2, Influenza, Hepatitis C virus and Coxsackievirus (Hober *et al*., 2014; Arena *et al*., 2018; El-Adawi *et al*., 2015; Mastromarino *et al*., 2011; Serkedjieva *et al*., 2000). However to the best of the author's knowledge, it is not known whether bacteriocins produced by lactobacilli species have antiviral activity against HIV as studies have mostly looked at bacteriocins from other bacterial species other than *Lactobacillus* (Férir *et al*., 2013). Ferir reported anti-HIV activity by a bacteriocin produced by *Actinomadura namibiensis*. **Figure 1.3** illustrates the various postulated mechanisms of lactobacilli protection against infections in the FGT.

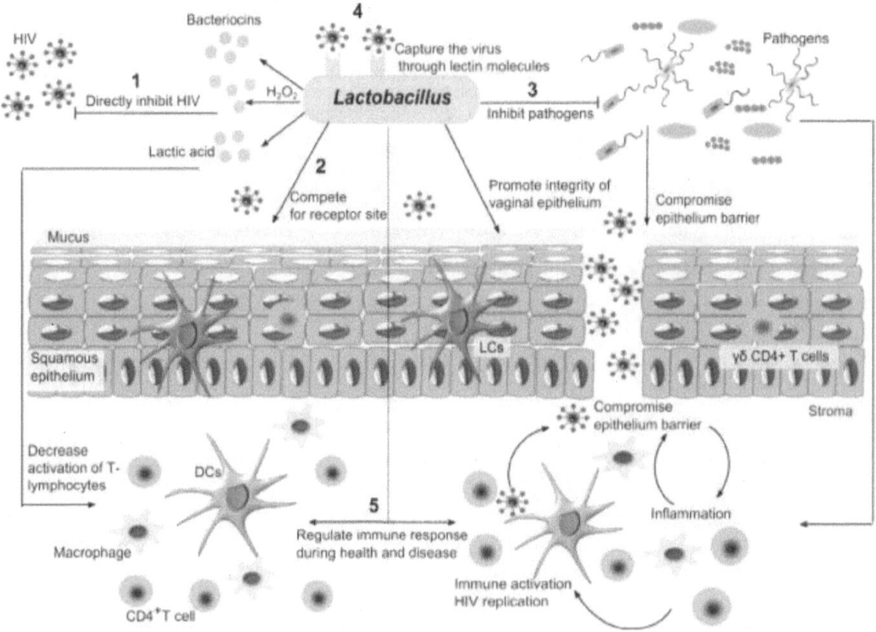

Figure 1.3: Protective mechanisms of *Lactobacillus* species in the female genital tract (FGT). (1) *Lactobacillus* species in the FGT can directly inhibit HIV by producing lactic acid, bacteriocins and H_2O_2. (2) Lactobacilli may also help maintain the integrity of the epithelium by competing for binding sites with pathogenic microorganisms. (3) Production of inhibitory compounds by lactobacilli can directly inhibit bacterial pathogens. (4) *Lactobacillus* species may also capture HIV via lectin-mediated binding to HIV glycoproteins and prevent productive infection during exposure. (5) Regulation and enhancement of the local immune system by lactobacilli. Vaginal lactobacilli may modulate local immune responses in the FGT during health or disease and therefore inhibit HIV acquisition. Figure adopted from (Petrova *et al.*, 2013).

1.4 Transmission of HIV across the cervicovaginal epithelial barrier

Normally, the likelihood of an exposure resulting in a productive HIV infection is very low due to a protective type II mucosa in the lower FGT (Miller *et al.*, 2005). Type II mucosae are characterised by multiple layers of non-keratinised stratified squamous epithelium with flattened surface cells and columnar cells in the deeper layer attached to the basal membrane (Robboy & Bentley, 2004). Potential mechanisms for HIV transmission across vaginal mucosal epithelium include (a) direct infection of epithelial cells; (b) transcytosis through epithelial cells or specialized microfold cells; (c) epithelial transmigration of infected donor cells; (d) uptake by intraepithelial Langerhans cells; (e) circumvention of the epithelial barrier through physical breaches. Successful transfer of the virus across epithelial barriers would result in viral uptake by migratory dendritic cells such as DC-SIGN or other mannose C-type lectin receptors and subsequent dissemination to T cells in the lymphatic system or localized mucosal infection, leading to recruitment of additional susceptible cells (Kwon *et al.*, 2002; Hladik *et al.*, 2007; Lederman *et al.*, 2006; Maher *et al.*, 2005; Pudney *et al.*, 2005; Stoddard *et al.*, 2010; Wu *et al.*, 2003; Hladik & Hope, 2019). **Figure 1.4** illustrates the postulated mechanisms for HIV transmission across the cervicovaginal mucosa.

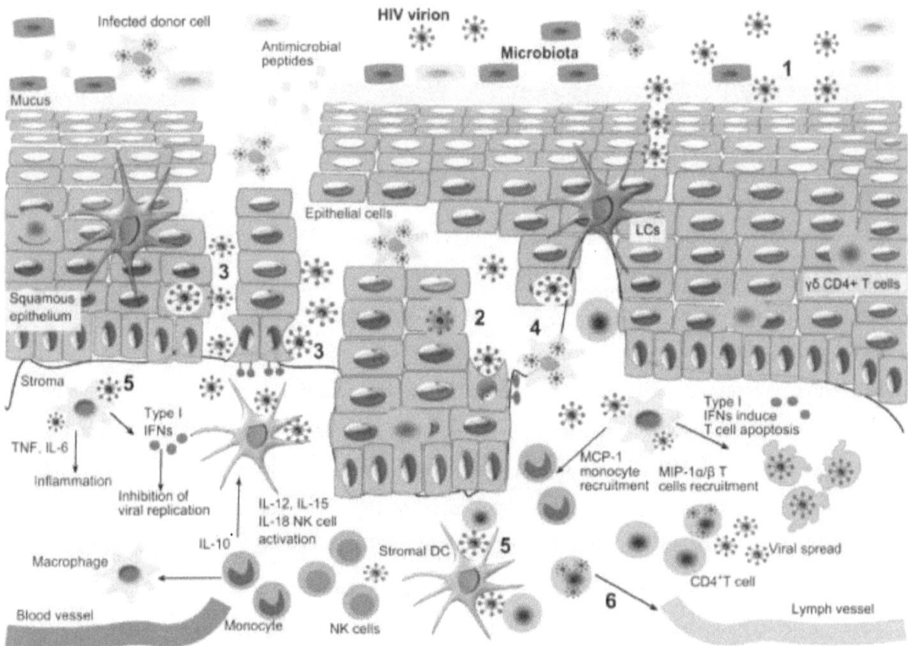

Figure 1.4: Postulated mechanisms for HIV transmission across the vaginal mucosa. The vaginal epithelium is covered by a type II mucosa. This type of epithelium is covered by a thick layer of mucus that provides a barrier against invading pathogens. Type II mucosae are characterised by multiple layers of non-keratinised stratified squamous epithelium with flattened surface cells and transforms into a single columnar layer in the deeper layer attached to the basal membrane. Innate immune cells including dendritic cells (DCs), Langerhans cells (LCs), $CD4^+$ T cells and macrophages are also located in this layer. HIV virions may invade this epithelium in various ways. (**1**) Free HIV virions trapped in the mucus layer can directly penetrate the epithelium via gaps between epithelial cells. Additionally, infected donor cells trapped in the mucus layer may release infectious virions. LCs located in epithelial layer may internalize the virions into their cytoplasmic compartment and transport them into the submucosa. (**2**) The HIV virions can directly infect $CD4^+$ T cells on the epithelium via receptors including CXCR4 and CCR5 co-receptor binding. (**3**) Transcytosis: Free HIV virions or virions that have been released from infected donor cells can be transported through the epithelium by transcytosis resulting in a productive infection of the cells. (**4**) Migration of virions into the submucosa. Infected donor cells or free HIV virions can be transmitted through a disrupted vaginal mucosa into the submucosa. (**5**) Viral uptake by local immune cells. Free HIV virions can directly infect stromal CD4+ T cells and macrophages. Virions may also make contact with DCs and subsequently be transported to $CD4^+$ T cells. (**6**) Spreading the HIV infection: Infected $CD4^+$ T cells, macrophages, DCs and LCs can transport the HIV virions into the submucosa and to the draining lymphatics. Figure adopted from (Petrova *et al.*, 2013).

1.5 HIV entry and replication

The HIV virus has three structural genes namely Gag, Pol and Env. The Gag gene encodes the core structural proteins including p24 and the Env gene encodes the viral envelope glycoproteins gp 41 and gp120, which are involved with the recognition of cell surface receptors (Weiss, 1993). The Pol gene encodes enzymes critical for replication of the virus, namely reverse transcriptase that converts viral RNA into DNA, integrase that incorporates viral DNA into host chromosomal DNA and protease that cleaves large Gag and Pol precursors into their components. (Takebe, 2001; Sarafianos *et al.*, 2009). The entry of HIV into host cells can be divided into three main events: virus binding to the cell, activation and fusion. The viral envelope complex, composed of the heterodimer proteins gp120 and gp41, is essential for virus recognition and entry into target cells such as CD4^{+} T cells (Rizzuto and Sodroski, 1997; Fanales-Belasio *et al.*, 2010). During entry into the host cell, HIV gp120 binds to the CD4+ receptor which functions together with chemokine coreceptors CXCR4 and CCR5 on the host cell membrane (Simon *et al.*, 2006). By forming pores, the virion fuses with the host cell through gp41-mediated membrane fusion and then the viral capsid is released into the cytoplasm (Simon *et al.*, 2006; Weissenhorn *et al.*, 1997). Thus, activated CD4+ T cells, monocyte/macrophage lineage cells, and dendritic cells (DCs) are the main target cells for productive HIV infection since these cells express both CD4 and CCR5 and CXCR4 co-receptors. Some subsets of memory CD4+ T cells such as Th 17 have been shown to be infected at higher rates compared to others (Cavrois *et al.*, 2017). Following entry, HIV-1 is reverse transcribed, producing complementary DNA which is incorporated into the host cell nucleus for integration as a provirus into the host genome using the viral integrase enzyme (Lawn *et al.*, 2001). The pro-viral DNA directs the synthesis and processing of viral proteins, which assemble to form an HIV virus particle (Simon *et al.*, 2006). The particle migrates to the host cell surface, acquiring a surface glycolipid envelop as it buds off and migrates to another susceptible host cell and undergoes the same process in another cell in the host (Lawn *et al.*, 2001; Simon *et al.*, 2006). The infected host cell dies during this process.

1.6 Factors that increase HIV acquisition risk

1.6.1 FGT inflammation and risk of HIV acquisition

The odds of HIV acquisition were increased 3.2-fold in women who had elevated levels of at least five pro-inflammatory cytokines, including macrophage inflammatory protein (MIP)-1α, IL-8, MIP-1β, IL-1β, IL-1α, monocyte chemoattractant protein (MCP)-1, IP-10, IL-6 and TNF-α in cervicovaginal lavage (Masson *et al.*, 2015). Additionally, upregulation of RANTES and downregulation of SLPI levels have also been associated with an increased risk of HIV acquisition in women (Morrison *et al.*, 2014). It has also been shown that upregulated inflammatory cytokines including IL-1α, IL-1β, IL-6, TNF-α, IL-8, IP-10, MCP-1, MIP-1α, MIP-1β were associated with abrogated efficacy of tenofovir microbicide gel suggesting that the presence of inflammation in the FGT may compromise HIV prevention efforts (McKinnon *et al.*, 2018).

Chemokines act as chemoattractants leading to the migration of immune cells to an infection site and downregulation may suggest subsequent reduction in target cell recruitment. In addition to recruiting and activating potential HIV target cells, pro-inflammatory cytokines activate the long-terminal repeat (LTR) promoter region of HIV-1 through the transcription factor nuclear factor kappa B (NF-κB) pathway, thus stimulating HIV-1 replication (Osborn *et al.*, 1989; Thurman & Doncel, 2011). NF-κB binds to the HIV LTR and induces HIV transcription. Persistent secretion of cytokines may additionally compromise the integrity of the mucosal surface (Svanborg *et al.*, 1999).

1.6.2 Non-optimal vaginal microbiota and risk of HIV acquisition

BV and non-optimal microbiota are characterised by the loss of *Lactobacillus* species and an overgrowth of strict or facultative anaerobic bacteria (Fredricks *et al.*, 2005; Hearps *et al.*, 2017). It is reported to be the most prevalent genital tract disorder in women of child bearing age and a substantial population of reproductive-aged HIV-uninfected women from different regions in South Africa, where HIV is also prevalent, have BV (Masson *et al.*, 2014). Some of the most common organisms associated with BV include *Gardnerella vaginalis*, *Prevotella* spp., *Mycoplasma hominis*, *Mobiluncus* spp., and *Atopobium* (Eastment & McClelland, 2018; Lennard *et al.*, 2017), although the composition of the vaginal microbiota may vary from one BV positive woman to another. The changes that occur in the FGT that are associated with BV include an increased vaginal pH (>4.5) and a vaginal discharge with a characteristic amine odor after addition of 10 percent potassium hydroxide to vaginal secretions (Cauci, 2004; Taha *et al*., 1998). Vaginal itchiness or burning may also be present, however studies have shown that approximately 40% of women with BV are asymptomatic (Klebanoff *et al*., 2004). BV is associated with increased susceptibility to HIV and STIs such as *Chlamydia trachomatis*, *Neisseria gonorrhoeae*, *Trichomonas vaginalis,* herpes simplex virus type 2 (HSV-2), and adverse reproductive health outcomes (Brotman *et al*., 2017; Cherpes *et al*., 2003; Haggerty *et al*., 2004; Ness *et al*., 2005; Rathod *et al*., 2012; Wiesenfeld *et al*., 2003). Furthermore, HIV-infected women with BV are over 3-times more likely to transmit HIV to their partners due to higher HIV RNA levels in the vaginal fluid as compared to the levels in women with optimal vaginal microbiota (Cohen *et al*., 2012; Cu-Uvin *et al*., 2001). In addition to the impact of BV on HIV, BV increases the risk of miscarriage, preterm labour, and postpartum complications such as endometritis and wound infections (Koumans *et al*., 2007).

The current treatment consists of oral and intravaginal doses of metronidazole or clindamycin (Bradshaw *et al*., 2006). BV is frequently recurrent following antibiotic treatment, the current standard of care and there have been reports of more than 50% of treated cases recurring within 6-12 months after treatment (Hillier *et al*., 1993). Due to the frequently asymptomatic nature of BV, the detection of cases poses a significant challenge (Klebanoff *et al*., 2004). The gold standard for BV diagnosis is by Nugent's criteria which involves Gram staining of vaginal smears and visualization of non-optimal bacteria in the absence of optimal *Lactobacillus* species (Nugent *et al*., 1991; Koumans *et al*., 2007). Amsel's criteria is used clinically and evaluates the presence or absence of clue cells, a white homogenous discharge, vaginal fluid pH > 4.5 and release of a fishy odor on addition of potassium hydroxide to a sample of vaginal secretions (Amsel *et al*., 1983). More recently, rapid and molecular diagnostic tests have also been used for BV diagnosis (Fredricks *et al*., 2005; Ravel *et al*., 2011; Fettweis *et al*., 2012; Srinivasan *et al*., 2012; Borgdorff *et al*., 2015; Zevin *et al*., 2016; Klatt *et al*., 2017; Gaydos *et al*., 2017; McClelland *et al*., 2018; Schwebke *et al*., 2018). However, the aetiology and clinical course of BV are not yet fully understood and further studies need to be carried out to investigate the underlying mechanisms.

BV is associated with high levels of inflammatory cytokines in the FGT, particularly in younger women (Deese *et al*., 2015). Higher levels of cervicovaginal pro-inflammatory cytokines including IL-1β, IL-6, IL-1β and TNF-α have been found in women with BV in comparison to women without BV (Deese *et al.*, 2015; Hedge *et al.*, 2006; Masson *et al.*, 2014; Thurman and Doncel, 2011). It was found that vaginal fluid from women with BV stimulates myeloid cells to secrete inflammatory cytokines, while vaginal fluid from women with optimal microbiota was less stimulatory, suggesting an association between the presence of inflammatory cytokines and the vaginal microbiota in women with BV (John *et al.*, 2007; Zariffard *et al.*, 2005). Other studies have also shown that the presence of non-optimal microbiota such as *Gardnerella vaginalis* or *Prevotella bivia* induced inflammatory responses *in vivo* and *in vitro* (Hummelen *et al.*, 2010; Santos *et al.*, 2018; Chetwin *et al.*, 2019). On the other hand, downregulation of some cytokines, particularly chemokines like IP-10, has also been associated with BV (Ryckman *et al.*, 2008; Masson *et al.*, 2014; Deese *et al.*, 2015). Most importantly, cytokine and chemokine concentrations have been shown to normalise after successful BV treatment making it essential to prevent and treat BV in our population (Thurman & Doncel, 2011; Joag *et al.*, 2018).

The mechanisms underlying the loss of microbial balance in the FGT that leads to the development of BV are not fully understood. Whether the depletion of lactobacilli or the over-growth of BV-associated bacteria occurs first remains to be determined. However, sensitive gene amplification assays have detected low levels of BV-associated bacteria in the FGTs of women with *Lactobacillus*-dominated microbiota, suggesting that overgrowth of the BV associated bacteria such as *G. vaginalis* leads to BV (Fettweis *et al.*, 2014; Jespers *et al.*, 2012). *G. vaginalis* produces a toxin known as vaginolysin that aids in adherence of the bacterium to the vaginal epithelium, while facilitating biofilm formation necessary for bacterial persistence and evasion of host defense mechanisms (Patterson *et al.*, 2010). On the other hand, *P. bivia* was shown to possess a strong capacity to invade HeLa cells *in vitro* and produce virulence factors, thus enabling the establishment of an upper genital tract infection (Strömbeck *et al.*, 2007). Additionally, antibiotic treatment, douching and sexual intercourse have also been associated with the loss of lactobacilli in the FGT, resulting in increased susceptibility to pathogens and an increase in diverse microbial populations (Rose *et al.*, 2012). Due to lack of competition, the pathogens are able to infect, causing BV and urogenital infections such as fungal vaginitis and STIs (Wiesenfeld *et al.*, 2003; Cherpes *et al.*, 2003; Brotman, 2011; Rathod *et al.*, 2012; Wagner *et al.*, 2012).

1.7 Regulation of the immune system by *Lactobacillus* species

Interestingly, cytokine profiles of vaginal epithelial cells were not affected after colonization with these *Lactobacillus* vaginal strains but studies have shown that lactobacilli regulate the immune responses in the FGT, which may ultimately prevent bacterial, viral and fungal infections (Cauci & Culhane, 2007; De Gregorio *et al*., 2016; Taweechotipatr *et al*., 2009; Hearps *et al*., 2017; Santarmaki *et al*., 2017). However, little is known about the underlying mechanisms. As mentioned above, BV is accompanied by an increase in inflammatory cytokines and has been shown to be associated with increased susceptibility to STIs including HIV (Cherpes *et al*., 2003; Eastment *et al*., 2015; Gillet *et al*., 2011; Lennard *et al*., 2017; Rathod *et al*., 2012; Wiesenfeld *et al*., 2003). Therefore, bacteria that can downregulate inflammatory responses may contribute to decreased HIV acquisition risk (Gosmann *et al*., 2017). Significant downregulation of TNF, MIP-1β and RANTES expression was observed in response to TLR agonists in vaginal multilayer systems pretreated with *L. crispatus* ATCC 33820 or *L. jensenii* ATCC 25258 (Rose *et al*., 2012). Additionally, *L. crispatus* ATCC 33820 significantly downregulated IL-6 and IL-8 (Rose *et. al*., 2012). *L. rhamnosus* GR-1 and *L. reuteri* RC-14 suppressed *C. albicans*-induced NF-kβ inhibitor kinase alpha (Ikkα), TLR2, TLR6, IL-8 and TNF expression, suggesting inhibition of NF-kβ signaling (Wagner *et al*., 2012). The anti-inflammatory effects of the lactobacilli were found to differ between agonists and strains, suggesting that the immune-modulating effects are strain-specific and depend on specific molecular interactions (Rose *et al*., 2012). Since NF-kB signaling results in increased replication of HIV and enhances progression of the infection, vaginal lactobacilli may also contribute to controlling HIV acquisition by suppressing NF-kβ (Wagner *et al*., 2012). Hearps *et al*. (2017) found that treating vaginal and cervical epithelial cells with lactic acid induced the production of IL-1RA, an anti-inflammatory cytokine, and inhibited the production of IL-6, IL-8, TNF-α, RANTES, and MIP-3α (Hearps *et al*., 2017). This suggests that lactic acid has an anti-inflammatory effect, further supporting the importance of FGT colonisation with lactobacilli in the context of HIV infection.

1.8 *Lactobacillus* species as a potential biotherapeutic in the FGT

Since the depletion or absence of lactobacilli in the FGT has been associated with development of BV in women (Hummelen *et al*., 2010), clinical trials have been carried out to investigate probiotic administration to recolonize the FGT with optimal *Lactobacillus* species. Probiotics are described as live organisms which can exert therapeutic benefits when administered in sufficient amounts (WHO, 2002). Probiotic bacteria may help prevent the high recurrence rates associated with the current standard of care and development of resistance to BV antibiotic treatment (Beigi *et al.*, 2004; Gupta *et al.*, 1999; Andreu *et al.*, 1995; Bradshaw *et al.*, 2006; Hemmerling *et al.*, 2010; Larsson *et al.*, 2008; Mastromarino *et al.*, 2002; Mastromarino *et al.*, 2009). To date, it has been shown that lactobacilli administered in the FGT are able to displace BV-associated pathogens and may help reduce HIV acquisition risk in women by restoring an optimal vaginal microbiota (Larsson *et al.*, 2008; Pendharkar *et al.*, 2013). Clinical trials have been conducted to assess the efficacy of orally or intravaginally administered probiotics on their own or as complementary treatment to antibiotics including metronidazole or clindamycin (Anukam *et al.*, 2006; Falagas *et al.*, 2007; Mastromarino *et al.*, 2009; Machado *et al.*, 2016; Eriksson *et al.*, 2005; Petricevic *et al.*, 2008; Bradshaw *et al.*, 2012; Hemalatha *et al.*, 2012; Ling *et al.*, 2013; Bisanz *et al.*, 2014; Verdenelli *et al.*, 2016; Bohbot *et al.*, 2018; Rapisarda *et al.*, 2018). Interestingly, the use of probiotics following antibiotic treatment has shown an increase in BV cure rate and reduced recurrence rates in some studies (Anukam *et al.*, 2006; Larsson *et al.*, 2008; van de Wijgert *et al.*, 2019). However, none of the trials have reported lactobacilli colonisation beyond the treatment period and it is therefore not clear whether the lactobacilli are able to persist well beyond the treatment period.

To improve persistence, probiotics may also be administered along with prebiotics to specifically stimulate the growth and colonisation of probiotic bacteria (Bouhnik *et al.*, 1997; Coste *et al.*, 2012; Gibson & Roberfroid, 1995; Rousseau *et al.*, 2005; Sutherland *et al.*, 2008; Vitali *et al.*, 2017). The ability of the lactobacilli to multiply in the FGT ensures an increase in size of the probiotic population. This, in turn, may increase the concentrations of protective metabolites secreted by the lactobacilli into the FGT such as lactic acid, increasing the beneficial effects. The characteristics of effective probiotics include the ability to adhere to vaginal epithelial cells and competitively exclude pathogens (Gueimonde *et al.*, 2006; Breshears *et al.*, 2015; Hütt *et al.*, 2016; Pendharkar *et al.*, 2013; Samuel *et al.*, 2016). The morphology of the lactobacilli has also been shown to play an important role, with the longer strains covering a greater epithelial surface area and therefore inhibiting adherence of pathogens (McLean *et al.*, 2000). The exclusion of pathogens is further facilitated by formation of a biofilm that covers epithelial cell receptors, preventing pathogen binding (Osset *et al.*, 2001). Production of lactic acid is also considered to be a critical probiotic-relevant property (Boris *et al.*, 1998; Boskey *et al.*, 2001), creating an acidic environment that inhibits pathogen growth in the FGT (O'Hanlon *et al.*, 2011; Aldunate *et al.*, 2013; Aldunate *et al.*, 2015; Tachedjian *et al.*, 2017; Tyssen *et al.*, 2018).

1.9 Study aims and objectives

The overall aim of this dissertation was to characterise the relative HIV inhibitory properties of vaginal *Lactobacillus* isolates, evaluate the immunomodulatory properties of the lactobacilli and to determine the mechanisms underlying these relationships. A better understanding of the immunomodulatory and other properties of vaginal lactobacilli is critical for the development of biomedical interventions to improve BV treatment and reduce HIV infection risk in women. As few studies have characterised vaginal *Lactobacillus* isolates in African populations, this study evaluated the influence of optimal vaginal *Lactobacillus* species isolated from South African women. This study included *Lactobacillus* species that are considered to be optimal and are associated with the lowest levels of inflammatory cytokine production *in vivo*, in order to further evaluate their immunomodulatory properties that may reduce HIV risk.

Specific objective 1

To describe the characteristics of vaginal lactobacilli isolates (including size, lactic acid production, adhesion, culture acidification, growth rates) and compare species and individual strains

Specific objective 2

To compare probiotic-relevant characteristics between vaginal lactobacilli isolates obtained from South African women and commercial vaginal probiotics available on the South African market.

Specific objective 3

To investigate the effect of lactobacilli conditioned culture medium on HIV pseudovirus entry in TZM-bl cells.

Specific objective 4

To evaluate the influence of vaginal lactobacilli on inflammatory responses in vaginal epithelial cells (VK2) to *Prevotella bivia* ATCC 29303 and *Gardnerella vaginalis* ATCC 14018

Specific objective 5

To compare the proteome profiles of vaginal inflammatory and non-inflammatory lactobacilli isolates

CHAPTER 2: MATERIALS AND METHODS

2.1 Study Cohort and sample selection

The *Lactobacillus* isolates analysed in this dissertation were obtained from cervicovaginal secretions collected from young women who participated in the European & Developing Countries Clinical Trials Partnership (EDCTP)-funded Women's Initiative in Sexual Health (WISH) study in Cape Town, South Africa (Principal Investigator: Associate Professor Jo-Ann Passmore; Barnabas *et al.*, 2018; Lennard *et al.*, 2017). The cohort study was conducted between June 2013 and March 2014 and comprised of 149 women (16-22 years). Ethical approvals to carry out the parent studies and this sub-study were obtained from the Human Research Ethics Committee (HREC) at the University of Cape Town (UCT HREC REF: 267/2013; UCT HREC REF: 551/2016 and UCT HREC REF: 267/2018, respectively).

2.2 Collection of demographic data and STI testing

Demographic data was collected from the women by questionnaire. Vulvovaginal swabs were collected for detection of STIs (HSV-1, HSV-2, *Mycoplasma genitalium, Trichomonas vaginalis, Neisseria gonorrhoeae*, *Chlamydia trachomatis* and *Treponema pallidum*) by nucleic acid amplification tests, while candidiasis and BV were assessed by Gram stain (**Appendix I**), microscopy and Nugent scoring performed at the National Institute for Communicable Diseases (NICD). Women with non-optimal microbiota [BV positive (Nugent scores ≥7) and intermediate microbiota (Nugent scores between 4-6)]; women who were BV negative had scores between 0-3. Prostate specific antigen (PSA) was measured by ELISA assays (Human Kallikrein 3/PSA Quantikine ELISA, R & D Systems, USA) that were carried out by Dr Shaun Barnabas and Dr Smritee Dabee.

2.3 *Lactobacillus* isolation from vaginal secretions

Cervicovaginal secretions collected using menstrual cups (Softcup®, Evofem Inc, USA) were each diluted 1:4 in phosphate buffered saline (PBS) (Sigma-Aldrich, USA) and vortexed. Thereafter, 350µl of 60% glycerol were added to 650µl of each diluted sample and then stored in a -80°C freezer prior to bacterial isolation. Lactobacilli were isolated by thawing the stored secretions and culturing each sample in 1.5ml of de Man Rogosa and Sharpe (MRS) broth (prepared as described in **Appendix I**) for the differential culture of *Lactobacillus* species. The cultures were incubated for 48 hours at 37°C under anaerobic conditions. Oxoid AnaeroGen^{TM} anaerobic gas generating sachets (Thermo Fisher Scientific, USA) were placed in sealed containers with the culture plates to create an anaerobic environment for culture incubation. The bacterial suspensions were sub-cultured by transferring 10μl onto fresh MRS agar plates (prepared as described in **Appendix I**) under the same culture conditions. Pre-screening of the isolates was performed microscopically by Gram staining (**Appendix I**) the lactobacilli. Bacterial colonies from plates showing mixed growth were carefully re-streaked on fresh agar plates; single colonies were picked using sterile toothpicks and incubated at 37°C overnight in MRS broth. Ten microlitres of the overnight cultures were re-streaked onto fresh MRS agar plates to obtain pure cultures. Matrix assisted laser desorption ionization-time of flight (MALDI-TOF), a technique that measures the unique protein profile of an organism, was conducted at the University of the Western Cape and at the French National Centre for Scientific Research by Dr Remy Froissart to identify the bacteria to species level. Each isolated bacterial species was then cultured in 1.5ml of MRS broth in Eppendorf tubes under anaerobic conditions for 48 hours at 37°C. After incubation, the tubes were centrifuged at 2500 rpm for 5 minutes before discarding 1 ml of supernatant. The samples were vortexed until the cultures were homogenous before adding 250μl of 60% glycerol, vortexed briefly and then stored at -80°C glycerol for downstream experiments.

In total, 210 bacteria were isolated from the vaginal fluid and stored in 60% glycerol (carried out together with Mrs Hoyam Gamieldien from the Division of Medical Virology, UCT). Among these, the following *Lactobacillus* species were identified: 22 *L. crispatus,* 1 *L. gasseri,* 44 *L. jensenii,* 8 *L. johnsonii,* 38 *L. mucosae,* 2 *L. plantarum,* 22 *L. ruminis,* 19 *L. salivarius,* 22 *L. vaginalis*, while 32 isolates were non-lactobacilli. From these, 16 isolates were selected based on the maximum number of isolates that could fit on a Luminex plate to investigate the impact of *Lactobacillus* isolates on inflammatory responses to BV-associated bacteria described in Chapter 6. A sample size of 16 lactobacilli isolates also allowed for comparisons between different species with equal representation of each lactobacilli species, with 4 isolates selected from each of the most common species including *L. crispatus*, *L. jensenii*, *L. mucosae* and *L. vaginalis.* Additionally, this allowed an equal representation of isolates obtained from BV positive and BV negative women, that is 8 isolates from BV positive and 8 from BV negative women. The other 64 isolates were selected based on a power calculation to determine the number of isolates required to demonstrate a significant difference in the inflammatory properties of isolates obtained from BV positive women and BV negative women. Since some of the women had multiple isolates of the same species, the 64 isolates were randomly selected such that there was only one of each species from each woman to prevent the inclusion of the same strain more than once. Another 23 isolates [*L. crispatus* (n=7), *L. gasseri* (n=1), *L. jensenii* (n=5), *L. mucosae* (n=4) and *L. vaginalis* (n=6)] were selected for comparison of probiotic relevant characteristics to commercial probiotics (**Figure 2.1**).

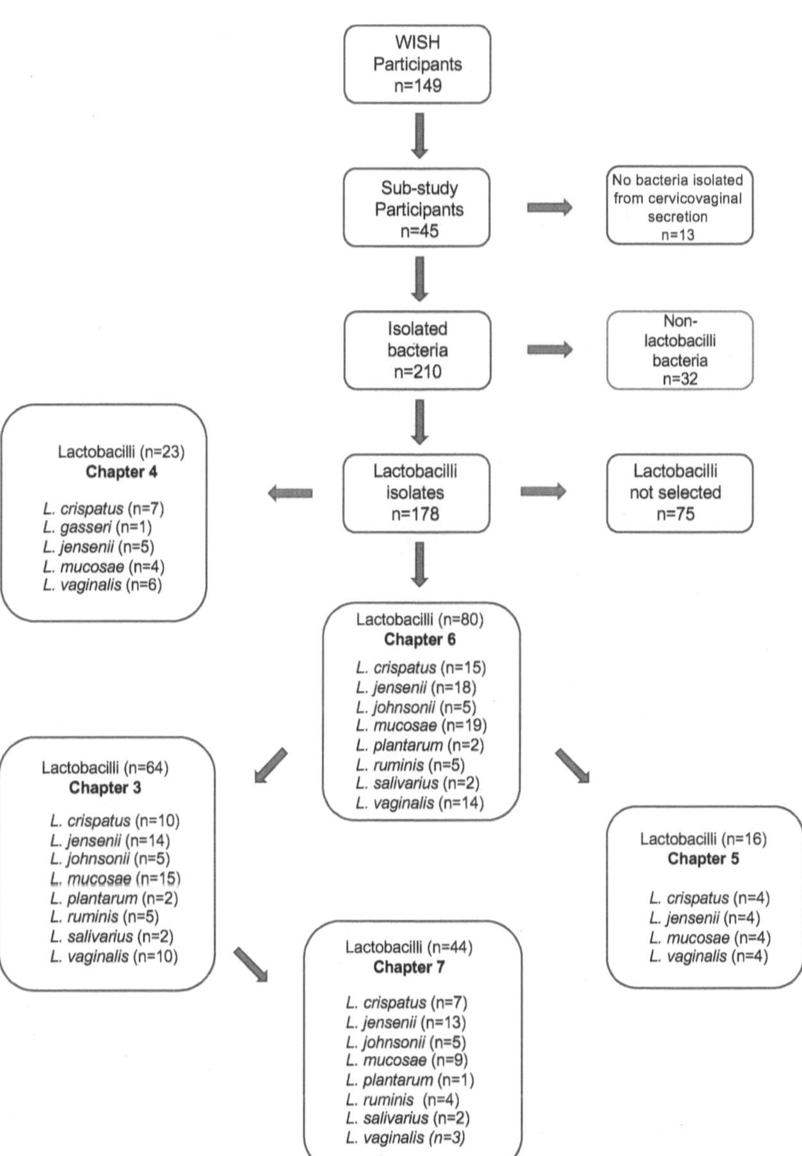

Figure 2.1 Flow diagram of the sequence of sample selection process for experiments.

2.4 Isolation of *Lactobacillus* species from commercial probiotics

Two commercial probiotics, Provacare and Vagiforte, were obtained from local pharmacies in Cape Town for comparison with vaginal lactobacilli. Vagiforte was supplied as vaginal pessaries and oral capsules, both containing *L. acidophilus*, *Bifidobacterium bifidum* and *Bifidobacterium longum* species. Provacare was supplied as vaginal capsules containing *L. casei rhamnosus*. The tablets were aseptically crushed and re-suspended in 1.5ml of MRS broth (prepared as described in **Appendix I**) before incubating for 48 hours at 37°C. To isolate single bacterial colonies, 10µl of the liquid cultures were streaked onto MRS agar plates (prepared as described in **Appendix I**) and incubated for 48 hours at 37°C under anaerobic conditions. To create an anaerobic environment, the plates were placed in tightly sealed containers with Oxoid AnaeroGen™ anaerobic gas generating sachets. The plates were carefully sealed using parafilm and sent for MALDI-TOF biotyping at the University of the Western Cape where the isolates were identified to species level as *L. casei rhamnosus* isolated from Provacare capsules and *L. acidophilus* isolated from Vagiforte tablets and capsules. *Bifidobacterium* species were not isolated for this dissertation.

2.5 *Gardnerella vaginalis* ATCC 14018 culture

The culture conditions for *Gardnerella vaginalis (G. vaginalis* ATCC strain 14018), one of the main BV-associated bacteria, were successfully optimized (carried out together with Dr Brian Kullin from the department of Molecular and Cell Biology, UCT). The *G. vaginalis* strain was supplied in a lyophilized form from ATCC and was revived in modified Brain Heart Infusion (BHI) broth (Sigma Aldrich, USA) prepared as described in **Appendix I** and then streaked onto Schaedler blood agar (Sigma Aldrich, USA; prepared as described in **Appendix I**), Columbia blood agar (Sigma Aldrich, USA) with 5% horse blood (**Appendix I**) or modified BHI agar. One set of the streaked plates were incubated in an anaerobic chamber and the other set in a tightly closed jar with Oxoid AnaeroGen™ anaerobic gas generating sachets placed in a 37°C incubator. Growth on the plates was then compared to determine the best media and culture conditions for optimal growth of the micro-organisms. BHI was selected as the best culture media for *G. vaginalis* growth and there was no marked difference in the number of colonies on agar between plates incubated in the anaerobic chamber and those incubated in a 37°C incubator. Glycerol stocks were prepared from the bacterial suspensions as described above and stored at -80°C for downstream experiments.

2.6 *Prevotella bivia* ATCC 29303 culture

The culture conditions for *Prevotella bivia* (*P. bivia* ATCC strain 29303*)*, the second BV associated bacteria analysed in this dissertation, was also successfully optimized. The lyophilized form of *P. bivia* was revived in Reinforced Clostridial broth (RCM; Sigma Aldrich, USA), streaked onto Brain Heart Infusion (BHI) and RCM agar plates (prepared as described in **Appendix I**). Two sets of BHI and RCM broth were also inoculated with *P. bivia* cultures for determination of optimal culture conditions in liquid medium. One set of the streaked plates together with one set of the liquid cultures were incubated in an anaerobic chamber and the second set of agar plates in a tightly closed jar with Oxoid AnaeroGen™ anaerobic gas generating sachets placed in a 37°C incubator. The lids on the second set of liquid cultures were tightly closed before placing the tubes in the 37°C incubator. The plates were then compared to determine the best media and culture conditions for optimal growth of *P. bivia*. RCM agar showed the best growth compared to the BHI agar and plates incubated in the anaerobic chamber showed better growth compared to the plates incubated in the 37°C incubator. However, there was no significant difference in growth between the liquid cultures incubated in the anaerobic chamber and those incubated in the 37°C incubator and downstream experiments in RCM broth were therefore carried out in the 37°C incubator. Glycerol stocks were prepared from the bacterial suspensions as described above and stored at -80°C for downstream experiments.

2.7 Culture concentration standardization and bacterial size

Lactobacillus isolates were grown from frozen stocks in 1.5 ml of MRS broth and incubated anaerobically for 24 hours at 37°C. The bacterial cultures were standardized to an optical density (OD) of 0.1±0.01 at a wavelength of 600nm. Serial dilutions of 1:100 were prepared for each bacterial isolate from the standardized cultures before being plated in duplicate onto MRS agar in 6-well plates. The plates were incubated for 48 hours at 37°C with Oxoid AnaeroGen™ anaerobic gas generating sachets (Thermo Fisher Scientific, USA). The colony forming units (CFU) were then manually counted. As each subsequent experiment required the addition of a consistent number of bacteria, the numbers of viable bacteria present in cultures with an OD of 0.1±0.01 were determined. These CFUs were used to quantify bacteria in downstream experiments by measuring the OD_{600} to determine the volume of culture needed for the addition of the required number of CFUs. This allowed for the standardisation of each culture prior to each experiment using spectrophotometry. For each isolate, single colonies were picked and smears were prepared on microscope slides. The slides were Gram stained and representative images were collected (Leica ICC50 HD, Leica Microsystems, Germany). Bacterial size was measured from images of the Gram stained slides taken at a 1000x magnification using Image J™ software. The mean of five measurements for each isolate was used for analysis.

2.8 Ca Ski cell culture

Complete cell culture media was prepared by adding fetal bovine serum (FBS; Thermo Fisher Scientific, USA) to a final concentration of 10% and penicillin and streptomycin (50U/ml penicillin, 50U/ml streptomycin; Sigma-Aldrich, USA) at a final concentration of 1% to Dulbecco's Modified Eagle's Medium (DMEM) with L-Glutamine (Sigma-Aldrich, USA). A frozen vial of human cervical epithelial cells, Ca Ski (CRL-1550, ATCC, USA), was gently agitated in a water bath set to 37°C for approximately 2 minutes to thaw the cells. The cells were then transferred to 8ml of prewarmed complete DMEM in a 15ml conical tube. The cells in medium were then centrifuged at 100x*g* for 2 minutes. The supernatant was discarded and the pellet of cells resuspended in 1ml of fresh complete DMEM before being transferred to a T25 cell culture flask with 7.5ml of prewarmed complete DMEM. Cells were incubated at 37°C with 5% carbon dioxide (CO_2) and checked for confluency using an inverted light microscope. At approximately 70-90% confluency, the cells were sub-cultured by removing media and washing with 5ml of PBS. In order to lift the cells, 1ml of 0.25% trypsin in 1mM EDTA (ThermoFisher Scientific, USA) was added and the flask was incubated for 10 minutes. The cells were observed under an inverted light microscope for detachment. When cells were completely detached, pre-warmed complete DMEM was added to the flask to inactivate the trypsin. The cells were then transferred to a 15ml tube and centrifuged at 100xg for 2 minutes. After removal of the supernatant, the cell pellet was then resuspended in 2ml of DMEM and counted using the Trypan blue exclusion method for downstream use (Santos *et al.*, 2018). For freezing, $2x10^6$ cells were resuspended in 1ml of cold freezing medium consisting of 85% DMEM, 10% FBS and 5% dimethyl sulfoxide (DMSO) (Sigma-Aldrich, USA), placed in a cryotube and placed in a Mr Frosty™ freezing container (ThermoFisher Scientific, USA) at -80°C. The cells were transferred to a liquid nitrogen storage container within 48 hours.

2.9 VK2 cell culture

Complete cell culture media was prepared by adding 44.1mg/L calcium chloride, 0.05mg/ml of bovine pituitary extract (BPE) (Sigma-Aldrich, USA), 0.1ng/ml human recombinant epidermal factor (EGF) (Sigma-Aldrich, USA) and 1% penicillin and streptomycin (50U/ml penicillin, 50U/ml streptomycin; Sigma-Aldrich, USA) to keratinocyte serum free medium (KSFM) (Sigma-Aldrich, USA) (Fichorova *et al.*, 1997). A frozen vial of human vaginal epithelial cells, VK2E6E7 (CRL-2626, ATCC, USA), was gently agitated in a water bath set to 37°C to thaw the cells. The cells were transferred to 8ml of a 1:1 mixture of DMEM and Ham's F12 (Sigma-Aldrich, USA) medium containing 10% FBS in a 15ml tube and centrifuged at 100xg for 7 minutes. The supernatant was discarded and the pellet of cells resuspended in 1ml of fresh complete KSFM before being transferred to a T25 cell culture flask with 7.5ml of prewarmed complete cell culture media. Cells were incubated at 37°C in 5% CO2 and checked for confluency using an inverted light microscope. At approximately 70-90% confluency, the cells were sub-cultured by removing media and washing with 5ml of PBS. A volume of 1ml of 0.25% trypsin in 1mM EDTA was added and the flask was incubated for 10 minutes. The cells were observed under an inverted light microscope for detachment. When cells were completely lifted, 8ml of 1:1 mixture of DMEM and Ham's F12 medium containing 10% FBS was added to the flask to neutralize the trypsin. The cells were then transferred to a 15ml tube and centrifuged at 100xg for 7 minutes. After removal of the supernatant, the pellet of cells was then either resuspended in 2ml complete cell culture medium and counted using the Trypan blue exclusion method for downstream use, or prepared for freezing. Passages were limited to a maximum of 15. For freezing, $2x10^6$ cells were resuspended in 1ml of cold freezing medium (85% DMEM, 10% FBS, 5% DMSO), placed in a cryotube and placed in a Mr Frosty™ freezing container (ThermoFisher Scientific, USA) at -80°C. The vials were transferred to liquid nitrogen storage within 48 hours for downstream experiments.

2.10 Determination of *Lactobacillus* growth rates

To determine the growth rates for each isolate, the *Lactobacillus* isolates were each cultured in 1.5ml of MRS broth in Eppendorf tubes and incubated at 37°C for 24 hours. After the incubation, each sample was standardized to $4.18x10^6$ CFU/ml in MRS broth as described in Section 2.6. Two hundred microlitres of each CFU adjusted bacterial suspension were transferred to a 96 well flat bottomed plate in triplicate and MRS broth was used as blank. The OD at a wavelength of 600nm was measured using a microplate spectrophotometer (Spectramax, USA) at 3-hour intervals from baseline up to 24 hours and these were used to calculate the area under the curve for each isolate during the exponential growth phase.

2.11 Qualitative adhesion of clinical *Lactobacillus* isolates to epithelial cells

Human vaginal epithelial cells (VK2/E6E7 ATCC® CRL-2616™) or Ca Ski cells, maintained in appropriate complete KSFM cell culture medium prepared as described above, were seeded into 8-well chamber slides (ThermoFisher Scientific, USA) at $1x10^4$ cells/well, incubated at 37°C with 5% CO_2 and grown to approximately 80% confluency. *Lactobacillus* isolates were cultured and adjusted to $4.18x10^6$ CFU/ml in MRS broth before being added to the VK2 or Ca Ski cell monolayers and incubated for 2 hours at 37°C with 5% CO_2. Non-adherent bacteria were washed off three times with sterile PBS. The chambers were removed from the slides according to the manufacturer's instructions and the slides were heat fixed then Gram stained. Representative images were then collected (Leica ICC50 HD, Leica Microsystems, Germany) and used to rank the level of adhesion for each isolate.

2.12 Measurement of cytokine production by VK2 cells

2.12.1 Stimulation of VK2 cells with vaginal *Lactobacillus* isolates, *G. vaginalis* and *P. bivia*

VK2 cells were seeded into 24-well tissue culture plates at $1x10^5$ cells/well and grown to approximately 80% confluency at 37°C in the presence of 5% CO_2. The cell culture medium was then removed and the monolayers gently washed with antibiotic-free culture medium. Lactobacilli cultures were each adjusted to $4.18x10^6$ CFU/ml as described in section 2.7, resuspended in 1 ml of antibiotic-free KSFM and added in duplicate to VK2-cell monolayers in culture and incubated for 25 hours (for *Lactobacillus* only stimulations) or 5 hours (for *Lactobacillus*-BV bacteria co-cultures) at 37°C under 5% CO_2. *G. vaginalis* ATCC 14018 cultures standardized to $1x10^7$ CFU/ml in antibiotic-free KSFM or *P. bivia* ATCC 29303 cultures standardized to $1x10^9$ CFU/ml (previously titrated by Miss Andrea Gillian Abrahams) were then added to the VK2 cell monolayers and plates were incubated for a further 20 hours at 37°C in the presence of 5% CO_2.

After the 20-hour incubation, culture supernatants were removed from each well, centrifuged at 15 000xg for 10 minutes and then stored at -80°C. VK2 cell-only, *Lactobacillus*-only *G. vaginalis*-only and *P. bivia*-only controls were included in duplicate on each plate as appropriate.

2.12.2 Measurement of cytokine concentrations in culture supernatants

Nine cytokines were measured in the bacterial/cell culture supernatants using a Magnetic Luminex® Screening Assay kit (R&D Systems, Inc., USA). The following pro-inflammatory cytokines and chemokines and anti-inflammatory cytokines were measured with a Human Premixed Multi-Analyte Kit: interleukin (IL)-6, IL-8, IL-1β, IL-1α, IFN-gamma-inducible protein (IP)-10, Macrophage inflammatory protein (MIP)-3α, MIP-1α, MIP-1β and IL-1 receptor antagonist (RA). Cell culture supernatant samples were thawed overnight on ice. Reagents provided by the kit manufacturers were warmed to room temperature prior to use. All reagents, standards and samples were prepared as per manufacturer's instructions. The supplied 25x wash buffer was diluted to a 1x solution using deionized water and standards were reconstituted in KSFM before a 3-fold dilution series was performed. The supplied microparticle cocktail was diluted in Diluent RD2-1 and vortexed gently before 50μl was added to each well of the 96 well microplate. Blanks, standards and samples (50μl) were added to appropriate wells in duplicate, sealed, wrapped in aluminium foil to protect the microparticles from light and incubated at room temperature on a horizontal orbital microplate shaker (800 rpm; Labnet Orbit P4, USA) for 2 hours. The microplate was subsequently placed on a magnetic plate washer for 2 minutes to allow the microparticles to be pulled to the bottom of the plate and washed 3 times with wash buffer using the appropriate wash-settings (Bio-Plex Pro™ Wash Station, Bio-RAD Laboratories, USA). Diluted Biotin Antibody Cocktail (50μl) was then added to each well before further incubation at room temperature on a horizontal orbital microplate shaker (800rpm) for 1 hour. The plate was washed as described above. Streptavidin-phycoerythrin diluted in wash buffer (50μl) was added to each well, incubated for 30 minutes at room temperature on the shaker and washed as described above. Wash buffer (100μl) was added to each well and incubated for 2 minutes on the shaker in order to resuspend the microparticles. A Bio-Plex Suspension Array Reader (Bio-Rad Laboratories, USA) was used to collect data. Standard curves for each analyte were generated using a five parameter logistic (5-PL) curve fit and sample concentrations calculated accordingly (BIO-Plex manager V4,

Bio-RAD Laboratories, USA). Any cytokine concentration below the detectable limit was assigned the value of the half of the lowest recorded concentration of that cytokine.

2.13 D- and L-lactate production by *Lactobacillus* isolates and pH changes

D- and L-lactate concentrations were measured in both *Lactobacillus* MRS culture and in *Lactobacillus*-VK2 or Ca Ski co-culture supernatants. For the evaluation of lactate production in MRS, each lactobacilli sample was cultured in MRS broth and incubated for 24 hours at 37°C under anaerobic conditions. After the incubation, each sample was adjusted to $4.18 x 10^6$ CFU/ml in 1ml of MRS broth and then incubated for a further 24 hours as above. The culture supernatant was collected from each sample and centrifuged at 15 000xg for 10 minutes before being stored at -80°C. For lactate measurement in bacterial-epithelial cell co-cultures, VK2 cells or Ca Ski cells were seeded at $1 x 10^5$ cells per well in 24-well tissue culture plates and grown to approximately 80% confluency at 37°C with 5% CO_2 in appropriate culture medium. Lactobacilli cultures were each adjusted to $4.18 x 10^6$ CFU/ml, resuspended in 1 ml of antibiotic-free cell culture medium, added to the VK2-cell/Ca Ski cell monolayers and incubated for 25 hours at 37°C under 5% CO_2. Culture supernatants were collected from each well and centrifuged at 15 000xg for 10 minutes. For lactate production in the presence of *G. vaginalis/ P. bivia,* lactobacilli cultures were each adjusted to $4.18 x 10^6$ CFU/ml, resuspended in 1 ml of antibiotic-free cell culture medium, added to the VK2-cell/Ca Ski cell monolayers and incubated for 25 hours at 37°C under 5% CO_2. Culture supernatants were collected from each well and centrifuged at 15 000xg for 10 minutes. The concentrations of D- and L-lactate in the culture supernatants collected from the MRS cultures and co-cultures were determined in duplicate using D-Lactate Colorimetric and Lactate Assay kits (Sigma-Aldrich, USA) according to the manufacturer's protocol. Optical densities were measured at 450nm for D-lactate and 570nm for L-lactate (Spectramax, USA) and values were converted to ng/µl against standard curve values, according to the manufacturer's instructions. Culture pH in the *Lactobacillus*-VK2 or Ca Ski co-culture systems was measured using Macherey-Nagel pH strips (GmbH and Co., Germany) and a pH meter (Jenway Bench pH Meter 2510, Bibby Scientific, UK) was used for *Lactobacillus* MRS culture supernatants. Total lactic acid was calculated using the Henderson-Hasselbach equation (O'Hanlon *et al*., 2013):

$$\mathrm{pH} = \mathrm{p}K_a + \log_{10}\left(\frac{[\mathrm{A}^-]}{[\mathrm{HA}]}\right)$$

The equation is based on the fact that protonated lactic acid (LAH), which is the microbicidal form of lactic acid rather than the lactate anion (LA-), is a function of both total lactate concentration (total lactate = D-lactate + L-lactate) and pH or hydrogen ions (H+) concentration as calculated using the pK_a of lactic acid (3.86).

2.14 Determination of HIV infectivity in the presence of clinical *Lactobacillus* isolates

2.14.1 HEK293T and TZM-bl cell culture

Human embryonic kidney (HEK293T) and TZM-bl cells were maintained in complete DMEM. Complete culture media was prepared by adding 1% pen/strep (50U/ml penicillin, 50U/ml streptomycin) and 10% FBS in DMEM. The cells were incubated at 37°C in the presence of 5% CO_2 and cells were observed under an inverted light microscope for confluency. The culture medium was replaced with fresh pre-warmed complete DMEM every 2-3 days. At approximately 80% confluency, the cells were lifted using 1ml of 0.25% trypsin in1 mM EDTA (ThermoFisher Scientific, USA) by first washing the cells in pre-warmed PBS and then incubating them in 1% trypsin for 3-5 minutes. When the cells were detached, the trypsin was inactivated by adding 8ml of complete DMEM and transferred to a 15ml conical tube before being centrifuged at 1000rpm for 3 minutes. After removal of the supernatant, the pellet of cells was then either resuspended in 2ml of DMEM and counted using the Trypan blue exclusion method for downstream use (Santos *et al.*, 2018) or split into two flasks with prewarmed complete DMEM. To prepare the cell suspension for cell counts, 10µl of cell suspension was mixed with an equal amount of trypan blue (Sigma Aldrich, USA) and the mixture placed onto a Neubauer chamber for cell counting. For cryopreservation, cells were resuspended in 1ml of freezing medium (85% DMEM, 10% FBS, 5% DMSO), placed in a cryotube and placed in a Mr Frosty™ freezing container (ThermoFisher Scientific, USA) at -80°C. The vials were transferred to liquid nitrogen storage within 48 hours.

2.14.2 Plasmid DNA preparation

Escherichia coli JM109 (Promega), used for the production of plasmid DNA, was harvested from an overnight culture in Luria-Bertani (LB) (Sigma-Aldrich, USA) broth (carried out by Riley Traviss from the Division of Medical Biochemistry and Structural Biology, UCT) and centrifuged at 6000x*g* for 15 minutes at 4°C. To harvest the plasmid DNA, PureYield™ Plasmid Midiprep kit (Promega, USA), which was supplied by the manufacturer with premixed buffers (P1, P2, P3, QC and QF), was used according to the manufacturer's instructions. The bacterial pellet was resuspended in 4ml of the first buffer P1 to lyse the bacterial cells containing the plasmid DNA. A second buffer P2 was added and mixed thoroughly before incubating at room temperature for 5 minutes. A third buffer P3 was added and mixed by vigorously inverting the tube about 4-6 times before being incubated on ice for 15 minutes. The tube was then centrifuged at 15 000x*g* for 10 minutes at 4°C. The supernatant was applied to an equilibrated Qiagen-tip and allowed to flow through by gravity flow. The Qiagen-tip was washed in buffer QC before eluting the DNA by applying buffer QF to the Qiagen-tip. The DNA was precipitated by adding isopropanol to the eluted DNA and mixed before centrifuging at ≥15 000xg for 30 minutes at 4°C. Thereafter, the supernatant was carefully decanted and the DNA pellet washed with 70% ethanol. The tube was then centrifuged at ≥15 000xg for 10 minutes before carefully decanting supernatant. The pellet was air-dried for 10 minutes and re-dissolved in 300µl of nuclease free water. The DNA was quantified using a NanoDrop spectrophotometer (Thermo Fisher Scientific, USA) with nuclease free water as a blank before being stored at -20°C for downstream use.

2.14.3 Preparation of HIV-1 env-pseudovirus

HEK293T cells were seeded at $4x10^4$ cells/well in 2ml of complete DMEM into a 6-well plate and incubated overnight at 37°C with 5% CO_2. When cells were about 40-60% confluent, 400µl of serum free and antibiotic free DMEM were aliquoted into 15ml conical tubes for each sample. In preparation for co-transfection of HEK293T cells, 3.2µl env DNA, 11.6µl PSG3 delta env and 22.5µl of polyethylenimine (PEI) were added to 400µl of DMEM and the mixture vortexed for 15 seconds before being incubated at room temperature to allow for complex formation. The HEK293T cells were co-transfected with the plasmid DNA, with the PEI acting as the transfection agent. The overlying media in the 6-well plates with the HEK293T monolayers was removed by suction and 1.5ml of pre-warmed fresh complete DMEM was added to each well. The PEI complexes were added to each well dropwise for even distribution. The plates were then swirled gently to mix the cells with PEI complexes and incubated at 37°C for 6 hours with 5% CO_2. The medium was removed and replaced with 2ml of fresh pre-warmed complete DMEM and incubated for 48 hours to allow for DNA uptake by the cells and expression of required protein. After 48 hours of incubation, the pseudovirus was harvested in the supernatant and filtered using 0.22μm filters before being stored at -80°C in aliquots of 600μl supplemented with FBS at a final concentration of 20%.

2.14.4 Chemiluminescent p24 ELISA for pseudovirus quantification

To quantify the harvested pseudovirus, a chemiluminescent p24 ELISA (Aalto Bio reagents, Ireland) was set up and a TROPIX detection system (Applied Biosystems, USA) was used. To coat the ELISA plates, 100μl of anti-HIV-1 p24 coating antibody diluted to 1:600 in sodium carbonate buffer were added to 96-well high bind assay plates (Whitehead Scientific, SA) and covered in aluminium foil then incubated overnight at room temperature. After 24 hours, the plates were washed 3 times with 100μl of tris-buffered saline (TBS) to remove unbound antibody. The plates were blocked by adding 100μl of 5% bovine serum albumin (BSA) (Biocom Biotech, SA)) to each well and incubated for 1 hour at room temperature. The BSA buffer in the ELISA plate was discarded and the plate was washed four times with 100μl of TBS. To inactivate the pseudovirus aliquots prepared above, 1% Empigen in TBS was added to the pseudoviruses and incubated for 1 hour and then the pseudovirus was serially diluted before adding 100μl to the antibody coated wells. Standards were prepared in duplicate by serially diluting a purified p24 protein (0-32 ng/ml) in 1% Empigen in TBS. The standards were added in duplicate and samples were added in triplicate to the 96-well plates into the appropriate wells. Blank rows were filled with 1x TBS to minimize evaporation and the plates were covered with aluminium foil then incubated at room temperature for 3 hours. The plates were washed 4 times with 1x TBS. Alkaline phosphatase conjugated mouse anti-HIV-1 p24 antibody (Aalto Bio reagents, Ireland) was diluted with TBS-0.1% Tween-20 (TBS-T) containing 20% sheep serum (Biocom Biotech, SA) and 2% BSA, and 100μl was added to each well then incubated for 1 hour. The plate was then washed 8 times in 1x TBS-T and twice with 1x TROPIX buffer to remove unbound antibody. The detection reagent, CPD-Star, was diluted 1:4 in TROPIX buffer and 50μl of the diluted reagent were added into each well, incubated for three minutes and then read on a Glomax® 96 Modulus Microplate luminometer (Promega, USA). Relative light units (RLUs) were used as an indication of luminescence.

2.14.5 Determination of HIV infectivity in the presence of clinical *Lactobacillus* isolates

To determine whether the vaginal *Lactobacillus* isolates influenced HIV pseudovirus infectivity, TZM-bl cells were seeded at $1x10^4$ cells/well in a 96 well tissue culture plate and incubated at 37°C with 5% CO_2 for 24 hours. Thereafter, 50μl of HIV pseudovirus (prepared as described above in section 2.14.4) was added in triplicate at a concentration of 200ng/ml in complete DMEM to the TZM-bl cells and incubated at 37°C with 5% CO_2 for 24 hours in the presence or absence of 10μl of conditioned lactobacilli culture medium. Control wells each containing 100μl of MRS broth and 50μl of pseudovirus were included in each experiment. A multichannel pipet was used to transfer 50μl of each sample to a 96 well opaque plate and Luminescence was read using a Glomax® 96 Modulus Microplate Luminometer (Promega, USA) to determine the quantity of the cells that were successfully infected by the pseudovirus and RLUs were used as an indicator of luminescence. The experiment was repeated 3 times.

2.15 Evaluation of *Lactobacillus* proteomic profiles

2.15.1 Preparation of *Lactobacillus* isolates for mass spectrometry analysis

The relative abundance of pre-defined lactobacilli proteins as identified by mass spectrometry was compared between inflammatory and non-inflammatory lactobacilli. The lactobacilli isolates were ranked according to inflammatory cytokine production by VK2 cells in response to each isolate determined by combining all proinflammatory cytokines and chemokines assessed onto one factor using principal component analysis (PCA) in STATA, generating a component estimate for each isolate and the scores were used to classify the lactobacilli as inflammatory or non-inflammatory. Thereafter, 22 isolates with the highest scores and 22 isolates with the lowest scores were selected to investigate differential protein expression between the two groups. *Lactobacillus* isolates were each cultured in 1.5ml of MRS broth and incubated anaerobically at 37°C for 24 hours. After the incubation, each sample was standardized to $1x10^{12}$ CFU/ml in MRS broth as described above in section 2.7. The Eppendorf tubes were centrifuged at 15 000xg for 10 minutes before discarding the supernatant making sure not to disturb the pellets at the bottom of the tubes. The bacterial pellets were each washed 3 times by adding 1ml of sterile PBS into each Eppendorf tube and centrifuging at 10 000rpm for 10 minutes before discarding the supernatant. The supernatant was removed and the bacterial pellets were sent for mass spectrometry analysis at the *Centre for Proteomic and Genomic Research* (CPGR) in Cape Town.

2.15.2 Protein extraction from *Lactobacillus* cultures and quantification

To extract protein from the *Lactobacillus* cultures, the pellets were resuspended in 100mM triethylammonium bicarbonate (TEAB) (Sigma, USA) 4% sodium dodecyl sulfate (SDS) (Sigma, USA) and sonicated for one minute. Thereafter, the samples were incubated at 95°C for 10 minutes. The samples were allowed to cool and nucleic acids were degraded by adding 250 units of benzonase nuclease (Sigma, USA) and incubating for 2 minutes at room temperature. The samples were then clarified by centrifugation at 10 000xg for 10 minutes at room temperature. Quantification of protein was performed using the Quanti- Pro BCA assay kit (Sigma, USA) according to the manufacturer's instructions.

2.15.3 On-bead hydrophilic interaction liquid chromatography digestion

To prepare the beads for the hydrophilic interaction liquid chromatography (HILIC) magnetic bead workflow, the HILIC beads (ReSyn Biosciences, SA) were aliquoted into a new tube and the shipping solution was removed. The beads were then washed twice with 250μl wash buffer [15% acetonitrile (ACN), 100 mM Ammonium acetate (Sigma, USA) at pH 4.5] for 1 minute. Thereafter, the beads were resuspended in loading buffer (30% ACN, 200mM Ammonium acetate pH 4.5) to a concentration of 5 mg/ml.

Freeze dried samples were resuspended in 200ml of MilliQ water. The samples were diluted in 50mM TEAB (Sigma, USA). A total of 50μg of protein from each sample was transferred to a protein LoBind plate (Merck, USA). Protein was reduced with tris 2-carboxyethyl phosphine (TCEP) (Sigma, USA) which was added to a final concentration of 10mM TCEP and incubated at 60°C for 1 hour. Samples were cooled to room temperature and then alkylated with methylmethanethiosulphonate (MMTS) (Sigma, USA) which was added to a final concentration of 10mM and incubated at room temperature for 15 minutes. HILIC magnetic beads were added at an equal volume to that of the sample and a ratio of 5:1 with the total protein. The plate was incubated at room temperature on the shaker at 900rpm for 30 minutes to allow for binding of protein to beads. After binding, the beads were then washed 4 times with 500µl of 95% ACN for 1 minute. Trypsin (Promega, USA), made up in 50mM TEAB was added at a ratio of 1:10 with the total protein for protein digestion and the plate was incubated at 37°C on the shaker for 4 hours. After digestion, the supernatant containing peptides was removed and dried down. Samples were then resuspended in liquid chromatography (LC) loading buffer made up of 0.1% formic acid (FA) and 2.5% ACN.

2.15.4 Liquid chromatography mass spectrometry protocol

Liquid chromatography tandem mass spectrometry (LC-MS/MS) analysis was conducted with a Q-Exactive quadrupole-Orbitrap mass spectrometer (Thermo Fisher Scientific, USA) coupled with a Dionex Ultimate 3000 nano-UPLC system. Data were acquired using Xcalibur v4.1.31.9, Chromeleon v6.8 (SR13), Orbitrap MS v2.9 (build 2926) and Thermo Foundations 3.1 (SP4). Peptides were dissolved in 0.1% FA (Sigma, USA), 2% ACN and loaded on a C18 trap column 300µm×5mm×5µm (Thermo Fisher Scientific, USA). Samples were trapped onto the column and washed for 3 minutes before the valve was switched and peptides eluted onto the analytical column as described below. Chromatographic separation was performed with a Waters nanoEase (Zenfit) M/Z Peptide CSH C18 column (186008810, 75µm×25cm×1.7µm) as described below. The solvent system employed included solvent A: LC water (Burdick and Jackson, USA), 0.1% FA and solvent B: ACN, 0.1% FA. A multi-step gradient (summarized in **Table 2.1** below) for peptide separation was generated at 300 nl/min as follows: time change 3 minutes, gradient change 2 – 6% Solvent B; time change 58 minutes, gradient change 6 – 16% Solvent B, time change 26 minutes, gradient change 16 – 30% Solvent B; time change 0.1 minutes, gradient change 30 – 95% Solvent B. The gradient was then held at 95% Solvent B for 10 minutes before returning it to 2% Solvent B. To ensure carryover did not occur between runs, a wash step was added at the end of each run which comprised a gradient change of 2 – 50% Solvent B in 25 minutes, this was run at 400 nL/min. The gradient was held at 50% Solvent B for 10 minutes before returning to 2% Solvent B and conditioning the column for 15 minutes. All data acquisition was obtained using Proxeon stainless steel emitters (Thermo Fisher, USA). The mass spectrometer was operated in positive ion mode with a capillary temperature of 320°C and the applied electrospray voltage was 1.95 kV.

Table 2.1: Multi-step gradient for peptide separation

Time (min)	Flow rate (µl/min)	Solvent A (%)	Solvent B (%)
0.00	0.300	98	2
3.00	0.300	98	2
6.00	0.300	94	6
64.00	0.300	84	16
90.00	0.300	70	30
90.10	0.400	5	95
100.00	0.400	5	95
100.10	0.400	98	2
125.00	0.400	50	50
135.00	0.400	50	50
135.10	0.300	98	2
150.00	0.300	98	2

2.16 Statistical analysis

Data was analysed using STATA™ Version 12 (StataCorp, College Station, Texas), GraphPad Prism version 7 (GraphPad software, San Diego, California) and R Version 1.1.447 (The R Foundation for Statistical Computing, Vienna, Austria). Distribution of variables was assessed by Shapiro-Wilk test. Mann-Whitney U test was used for unmatched comparisons and Spearman Rank test was used to test for correlations for non-parametric data. Kruskal-Wallis tests were used to compare characteristics between different lactobacilli species. Fisher's exact test was used to compare proportions. Unsupervised hierarchical clustering was used to evaluate overall cytokine production by VK2 cells in response to lactobacilli stimulations. Multivariate linear and logistic regression analyses were used to adjust for possible confounders. A false discovery rate (FDR) step-down procedure was used to adjust p-values for multiple comparisons, with adjusted p-values <0.05 being considered statistically significant.

A scoring system was developed in order to compare probiotic relevant characteristics between vaginal lactobacilli, ATCC reference strains and commercial probiotics. The characteristics scored included culture acidification (3 points), lactic acid production (3 points), adhesion to Ca Ski cells, growth rates (3 points) and size (3 points). Each of the characteristics was scored according to specific criteria. For quantitative adhesion, isolates that showed $\geq$ 2% adhesion to Ca Ski cells were assigned a score of 6, isolates showing $\geq$ 0.5% <2% adhesion scored 4 points and those showing < 0.5% scored 2 points. Culture pH between 3.5$\leq$4 scored 3 points, pH between >4 $\leq$4.5 scored 2 points, between 4.5 $\leq$5 scored 1 point and culture pH greater than 5 scored 0 points. Relative scores for lactobacilli adhesion to Ca Ski cells, D and L-lactate production, growth rates and size were assigned as follows: $\leq$25th percentile (score = 0); 25th $\leq$ 50th percentile (score = 1); 50th $\leq$ 75th percentile score = 2); $\geq$75th (score = 3). The level of lactobacilli adhesion to VK2 cells was scored (1-6) by two individuals with least adherent isolate being given a score of 1 and the most adherent scoring 6.

Extracted LC-MS/MS spectra were searched against a UniProt sub-database including the *Lactobacillus* genus, as well as common contaminants, using the Andromeda search engine in MaxQuant version 1.5.7.4. The MaxQuant parameters for protein identification are shown in **Table 2.2**. Protein relative abundance was estimated using intensity-based absolute quantification (iBAQ). Protein functions were determined using aggregated gene ontologies (GOs) from UniProt and taxonomy was assigned using UniProt and the transformed iBAQ values of proteins with same assigned taxa for each sample were then aggregated. Differentially abundant proteins and GOs were identified using the linear models for microarray data (limma) R package. Protein functions were compared between lactobacilli inducing low levels of inflammatory cytokine production and lactobacilli inducing high levels of inflammatory cytokine production by VK2 cells. PCA was used to cluster lactobacilli according to species and inflammatory profiles using the mixOmics package in R. Clustering of lactobacilli according to the relative abundance of differentially abundant proteins was generated by unsupervised hierarchical clustering in R. Spearman correlations between differentially abundant proteins and lactobacilli characteristics such as adhesion and lactate production were determined in STATA. Logistic and linear regression analyses were used to adjust for confounders, including batch number and species, in STATA.

Table 2.2. MaxQuant parameters for protein identification

MaxQuant Parameter	Value/Description
Version	1.5.7.4
Fixed modifications	Carbamidomethyl (C)
Enzyme	Trysin/P
Include contaminants	TRUE
PSM FDR	0.01
Protein FDR	0.01
Site FDR	0.01
Use Normalized Ratios For Occupancy	TRUE
Min. unique peptides	0
Min. razor peptides	1
Min. peptides	1
Modifications included in protein quantification	Oxidation (M);Acetyl (Protein N-term)
Discard unmodified counterpart peptides	TRUE
iBAQ	TRUE
iBAQ log fit	TRUE
Decoy mode	revert
Include contaminants	TRUE
Second peptides	TRUE
Stabilize large LFQ ratios	TRUE
Require MS/MS for LFQ comparisons	TRUE
Min. peptide length for unspecific search	8
Max. peptide length for unspecific search	25
Razor protein FDR	TRUE

CHAPTER 3: Characteristics of cervicovaginal *Lactobacillus* isolates obtained from South African women

3.1 Summary

Bacterial vaginosis (BV) is a highly prevalent dysbiosis of the vaginal microbiota that puts women at an increased risk of HIV acquisition and adverse reproductive health outcomes compared to women without BV. The current standard-of-care is antibiotic treatment but complementary strategies to recolonize the FGT with *Lactobacillus* species are being investigated to improve treatment outcomes. Since different *Lactobacillus* species may vary in their capacity to protect the FGT from colonisation by bacterial pathogens, lactobacilli were isolated from the FGTs of South African women, identified to species level and characteristics considered important for vaginal colonization and competitive exclusion of bacterial pathogens were evaluated *in vitro.* Vaginal *Lactobacillus* isolates (n=64), including [*L. crispatus* (n=11), *L. jensenii* (n=14), *L. johnsonii* (n=5), *L. mucosae* (n=15), *L. plantarum* (n=2), *L. ruminis* (n=5), *L. salivarius* (n=2), *L. vaginalis* (n=10)] were isolated from young women and identified to species level using MALDI-TOF biotyping. Growth rates, bacterial sizes, adhesion to vaginal epithelial cells (VK2), culture pH changes and D/L-lactate production by the lactobacilli were also evaluated *in vitro* and compared among the lactobacilli isolates. It was found that these characteristics were highly varied both within and between species although no particular species appeared to markedly outperform the others when all characteristics were collectively evaluated. Total lactic acid and D-lactate production differed significantly between isolates obtained from women with optimal microbiota and those obtained from women with non-optimal microbiota. *L. jensenii* species was more frequently isolated in women with optimal microbiota. The presence of an STI or semen contamination was associated with the size or species of lactobacilli isolated from the women and bacterial size was inversely associated with semen contamination. In conclusion, the findings in this Chapter highlight the importance of thoroughly screening large numbers of species and strains obtained from different women to identify the best performing strains for probiotic development as there seems to be a large amount of variation in protective characteristics.

3.2 Introduction

BV is characterised by an alteration in the vaginal microbiota resulting from the depletion of *Lactobacillus* species and an overgrowth of non-optimal microbiota including diverse facultative and strict anaerobic bacteria such as *Gardnerella vaginalis, Prevotella* spp., *Mobiluncus* spp. and *Mycoplasma hominis* (Fredricks *et al.*, 2005; Eastment *et al.*, 2015; Lennard *et al.*, 2017). BV is one of the most common vaginal conditions in young women, although prevalence varies according to race and ethnicity for reasons that are not yet clear (Zhou *et al.*, 2007; Koumans *et al.*, 2007; Ravel *et al.*, 2011). Additionally, women with BV are at an increased risk of HIV acquisition and adverse reproductive health outcomes compared to women without BV (Hillier *et al.*, 1995; Taha *et al.*, 1998; Brotman *et al.*, 2011). The majority of women with BV are asymptomatic while other women present with a malodorous thin vaginal discharge (Klebanoff *et al.*, 2004; Koumans *et al.*, 2007). The diagnosis of BV can be based on clinical criteria or by Nugent scoring of Gram stained slides of vaginal fluid in the laboratory (Amsel *et al.*, 1983; Burton *et al.*, 2002). The current standard-of-care is antibiotic treatment but, due to high recurrence rates associated with this treatment strategy, probiotics have been used to complement antibiotic treatment by recolonizing the FGT with lactobacilli species (Gueimonde *et al.*, 2006; Sanders, 2008; Bradshaw *et al.*, 2006; Anukam *et al.*, 2006; Mohanty *et al.*, 2010; Homayouni *et al.*, 2013).

Lactobacillus species play a major role in the maintenance of vaginal health and are protective against genital infections/conditions such as BV, UTIs, vaginal candidiasis and STIs, including HIV (Gillet *et al.*, 2011; Aldunate *et al.*, 2013; De Gregorio *et al.*, 2016; Hütt *et al.*, 2016; Hearps *et al.*, 2017; Tyssen *et al.*, 2018). The most common lactobacilli species that have been isolated from the FGT include *L. iners, L. gasseri, L. plantarum, L. crispatus, L. rhamnosus, L. vaginalis, L. johnsonii, L. fermentum and L. jensenii* (Antonio *et al.*, 1999; Burton *et al.*, 2003; Tamrakar *et al.*, 2007; Ravel *et al.*, 2011). Although *L. crispatus* has been the most common species associated with health in the FGT, it is less frequently isolated from South African women compared to American or European women (Fettweis *et al.*, 2014; Zhou *et al.*, 2007; Anahtar *et al.*, 2015; Klatt *et al.*, 2017; Lennard *et al.*, 2017). Interestingly, while *L. iners* is often isolated from asymptomatic South African women, the role played by this species in vaginal health is still not well understood since it is present in women with a low diversity microbiome and low levels of inflammatory cytokines in the FGT (Burton & Reid, 2002; Srinivasan *et al.*, 2012), as well as women with non-optimal microbiota (Verstraelen *et al.*, 2009; Shi *et al.*, 2009; Tärnberg *et al.*, 2002; Verhelst *et al.*, 2004; Zhou *et al.*, 2004). Additionally, the species has been associated with upregulation of inflammatory cytokine production in vaginal epithelial cells (Doerflinger *et al.*, 2014). It is therefore not clear if *L. iners* dominance should be considered healthy in South African women. Lactobacilli are thought to protect against pathogens due to their ability to produce antimicrobial substances such as lactic acid and bacteriocins (Aroutcheva *et al.*, 2001; Atassi *et al*, 2006; Hearps *et al.*, 2017; Tachedjian *et al.*, 2017). While the majority of *Lactobacillus* spp. produce both D- and L-lactic acid, *L. iners* produces only L-lactic acid (Witkin *et al.*, 2013). Lactic acid maintains the vaginal pH below 4.5 and therefore creates an inhibitory environment for the growth of pathogens, including HIV (Aldunate *et al.*, 2013; Tachedjian *et al.*, 2017). Bacteriocins are proteins that are produced by lactobacilli that have bactericidal activity and are able to inhibit the growth of a diverse group of pathogenic bacteria, including *G. vaginalis* (Mclean *et al.*, 2000; Hütt *et al.*, 2016). Although it was initially thought that H_2O_2 production by lactobacilli conferred protection in the FGT (Hawes *et al.*, 1996; Klebanoff *et al.*, 1991; Sgibnev *et al.*, 2015), it has been shown that lactobacilli do not produce large amounts of H_2O_2 under anaerobic conditions, that are similar to those found in the vagina, compared to aerobic conditions (Ocana.,1999). This suggests that H_2O_2 produced in the vagina may not be microbicidal (O'Hanlon *et al.*, 2011). Additionally, when H_2O_2 was added to *in vitro* cultures at microbicidal concentrations, lactobacilli were inactivated more effectively compared to BV-associated bacteria (O'Hanlon *et al.*, 2011). In addition, the ability of lactobacilli to adhere to the vaginal epithelium enables the competitive exclusion of pathogen binding (Osset *et al.*, 2001; Reid *et al.*, 2001; Heinemann *et al.*, 2000; Hütt *et al.*, 2006).

Although lactobacilli have been shown to have protective properties, different *Lactobacillus* species may vary in their capacity to protect the FGT from colonisation by bacterial pathogens (Osset *et al.*, 2001; Sanders, 2008; Verstraelen *et al.*, 2009). Additionally, it has been shown that probiotic properties are species and strain specific (Sanders, 2008), highlighting the importance of evaluating the properties of individual lactobacilli strains. In this Chapter, lactobacilli were isolated from the FGTs of South African women, identified to species level and characteristics considered important for vaginal colonization and competitive exclusion of bacterial pathogens were evaluated *in vitro.* As previous studies describing the differences in bacterial characteristics between *Lactobacillus* spp., both those isolated from probiotics and vaginal isolates, were carried out in other regions of the world, including the USA and Europe (Osset *et al.*, 2001; Sanders, 2008; Verstraelen *et al.*, 2009; Anukaml *et al.*, 2009; De Seta *et al.*, 2014; Hu *et al.*, 2013; Davar *et al.*, 2016), one of the aims of this dissertation was to compare key properties among lactobacilli from African women. The characteristics of lactobacilli species, including adhesion to vaginal epithelial cells, morphology/sizes and growth rates, were compared between individual lactobacilli isolates and species. Additionally, *Lactobacillus* properties were compared between women with optimal microbiota (BV negative) and women with non-optimal microbiota (intermediate and BV positive) in order to evaluate whether particular characteristics influence the ability of non-optimal microbes to colonize the FGT.

3.3 Methods

Cervicovaginal secretions were collected from young South African women who participated in the Women's Initiative in Sexual Health (WISH) study. Vaginal *Lactobacillus* isolates (n=64), including *L. crispatus*, *L. jensenii*, *L. johnsonii*, *L. mucosae*, *L. plantarum*, *L. ruminis*, *L. salivarius* and *L. vaginalis*, were isolated from the cervicovaginal secretions and identified to species level using MALDI-TOF biotyping as described in Chapter 2. Gram stains were prepared from the lactobacilli cultures before collecting images to determine the average bacterial size for each isolate using Image J^{TM} software. Growth rates for each isolate were determined by measuring the OD of cultures over time, (Chapter 2, section 2.9). The level of *Lactobacillus* adhesion to vaginal epithelial cells (VK2/E6E7) was determined by incubating the isolates with VK2 cell monolayers for 2 hours. The cells were then washed three times with PBS to remove unbound bacteria, Gram-stained and images were collected for scoring of the levels of adhesion. Culture pH changes were measured using a pH meter and D- and L-lactate production were measured using ELISA as described in Chapter 2.

3.4 Results

3.4.1 Study population

The 64 vaginal *Lactobacillus* isolates included in this analysis were obtained from 25 women who participated in the WISH study in Cape Town (Barnabas *et al.*, 2018). Twenty eight isolates were obtained from 13 women with non-optimal microbiota [8 BV positive women (n=20 isolates) and 5 women with intermediate microbiota (n=8 isolates)], and 36 isolates from 12 women with optimal microbiota. Demographic data are shown in **Table 3.1**. The median age of the women was 18 (range 16-22) years and all of the women were using hormonal contraceptives at the time of sample collection.

Table 3.1. Demographic and clinical characteristics of study participants

Clinical and laboratory findings	Optimal N =12 n (%)	Intermediate microbiota N =5 n (%)	BV positive N =8 n (%)
Black race	12 (100)	5 (100)	8 (100)
Median age in years (range)	18 (16-20)	20 (16-22)	17 (16-22)
Chlamydia trachomatis (PCR positive)	3 (25)	0 (0)	2 (25)
Neisseria gonorrhoeae (PCR positive)	3 (25)	0 (0)	0 (0)
Trichomonas vaginalis (PCR positive)	0 (0)	0 (0)	0 (0)
Mycoplasma genitalium (PCR positive)	0 (0)	0 (0)	0 (0)
HSV-2 IgG	0 (0)	0 (0)	0 (0)
HSV (PCR positive)	0 (0)	0 (0)	0 (0)
Treponema pallidum (RPR>1:4, TPHA positive)	0 (0)	0 (0)	0 (0)
Yeast cells	0 (0)	0 (0)	0 (0)
PSA positive	1 (8)	1 (20)	4 (50)
DMPA	3 (25)	1 (20)	0 (0)
Nur-Isterate	8 (67)	4 (80)	5 (63)
Implanon	1 (8)	0 (0)	3 (38)

BV, bacterial vaginosis; PCR, polymerase chain reaction; HSV-2, herpes simplex virus type 2; RPR, rapid plasma reagin; TPHA, Treponema pallidum hemagglutination; PSA, prostate specific antigen; DMPA, depot medroxyprogesterone acetate.

Five of the women had *C. trachomatis* infections and two had *N. gonorrhoeae* infections. None of the participants tested positive for *T. pallidum* or *T. vaginalis,* none were shedding HSV-2 and none had yeast infections.

3.4.2 Bacterial isolation and phenotypic characterisation of vaginal *Lactobacillus* isolates

3.4.3.1 Standardisation of bacterial cultures

The 64 isolates were identified as 8 different species [*L. crispatus* (n=11), *L. jensenii* (n=14), *L. johnsonii* (n=5), *L. mucosae* (n=15), *L. plantarum* (n=2), *L. ruminis* (n=5), *L. salivarius* (n=2), *L. vaginalis* (n=10)]. As each experiment required the addition of a consistent number of bacteria, the numbers of viable bacteria present in cultures with an OD of 0.1$\pm$0.01 were determined. Determining the numbers of viable bacteria present in cultures with an OD of 0.1$\pm$0.01 allowed for the standardisation of each culture prior to each experiment using spectrophotometry. All of the samples analysed were viable as growth was observed on all MRS agar plates. There was marked variation in CFUs/ml of cultures standardised to OD 0.1$\pm$0.01, both within and between different species with a range between 3.95×10^5 CFU/ml for an *L. crispatus* isolate to 5.00×10^{12} CFU/ml for an *L. vaginalis* isolate, suggesting large variation in the sizes of the isolates (**Figure 3.1A**). This data was used to standardise the cultures for all subsequent experiments. Collectively, *L. jensenii* isolates had the highest number of CFUs while *L. johnsonii* isolates had the lowest (**Figure 3.1B**).

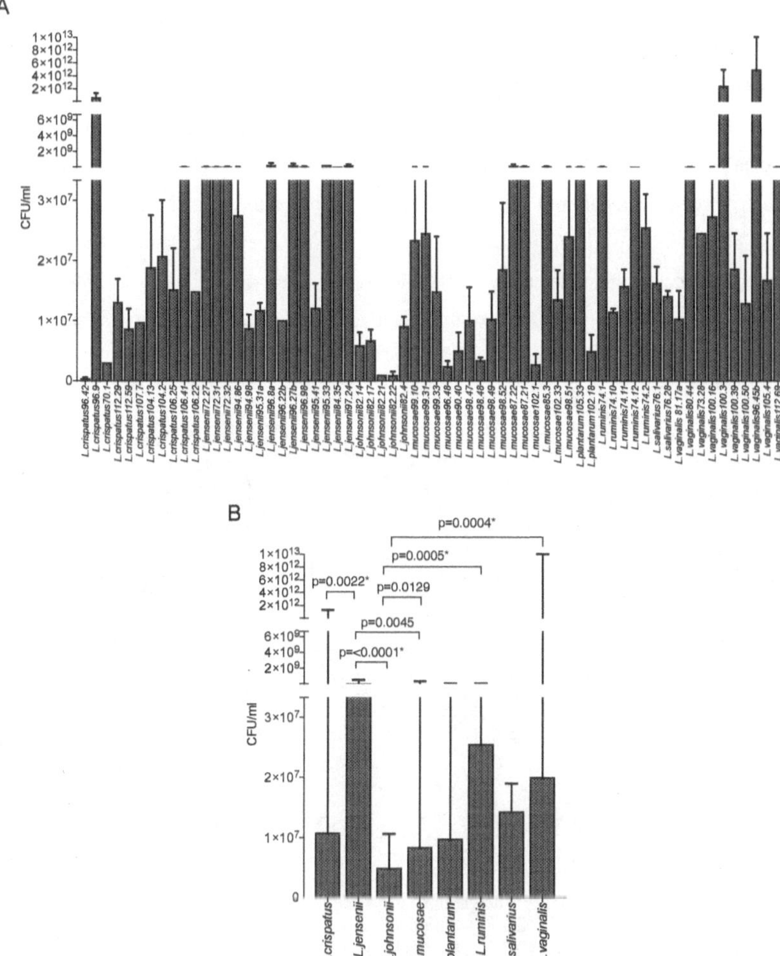

Figure 3.1: Number of colony forming units (CFU) of vaginal *Lactobacillus* cultures standardized to an optical density (OD) at 600nm of 0.1±0.01. (**A**) Lactobacilli CFU/ml for individual lactobacilli isolates with the species names and strain numbers labelled on the X-axis. Data are shown as medians with ranges. (**B**) Lactobacilli (CFU/ml) grouped by species including *L.crispatus* (n=11), *L. jensenii* (n=14), *L. johnsonii* (n=5), *L. mucosae* (n=15), *L. plantarum* (n=2), *L. ruminis* (n=5), *L. salivarius* (n=2), *L. vaginalis* (n=10). Lactobacilli were cultured in de Man Rogosa and Sharpe (MRS) broth, adjusted to an OD_{600} 0.1±0.01, serially diluted and then plated on MRS agar plates in triplicate. Following incubation for 24 hours under anaerobic conditions, CFUs were manually counted and CFU/ml calculated for each isolate. Kruskal-Wallis tests were used to compare CFUs between different lactobacilli species and p-values were adjusted for multiple comparisons using a false discovery rate step-down procedure. Adjusted $p<0.05$ were considered significant. *P values that remained significant after adjustment for multiple comparisons.

3.4.4 *Lactobacillus* morphology and bacterial sizes

To evaluate the morphological characteristics of the vaginal *Lactobacillus* isolates, the bacteria were cultured in MRS broth before being sub-cultured onto MRS agar plates and incubated anaerobically at 37°C for 48 hours. All the lactobacilli colonies appeared creamy or milky white, round and opaque when cultured on MRS agar plates, as previously described (Jose *et al.*, 2015). When single colonies were smeared onto microscope slides, heat fixed and Gram stained, the bacteria appeared as purple rods under a light microscope, as expected for Gram positive bacteria. **Figure 3.2 A-H** and **Appendix II** show representative images taken from the Gram stained slides with *Lactobacillus* isolates.

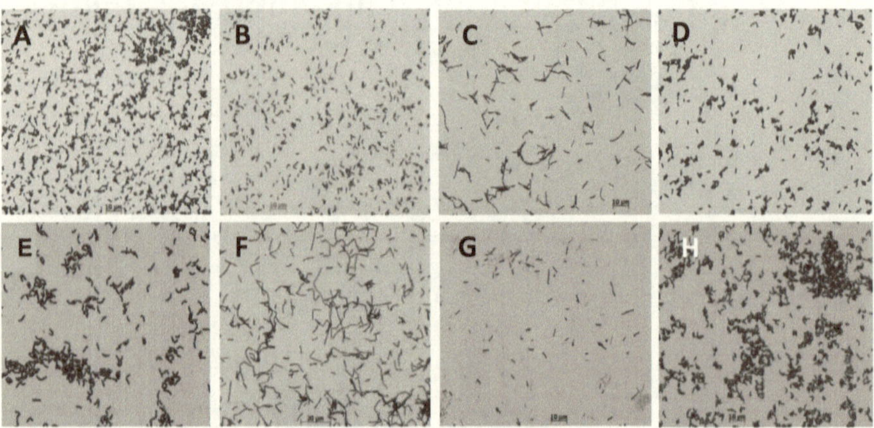

Figure 3.2: Gram stained images showing *Lactobacillus* morphology. *L. crispatus*106.25 (**A**), *L. vaginalis*81.17 (**B**), *L. ruminis74.10* (**C**), *L. johnsonii*82.22 (**D**), *L. mucosae*98.47 (**E**), *L. jensenii*96.9 (**F**), *L. salivarius*76.28 (**G**) and *L. plantarum*102.18 (**H**). Lactobacilli were cultured on de Man Rogosa and Sharpe (MRS) agar plates and incubated anaerobically at 37°C. Single colonies were picked from each plate and smeared onto glass slides before preparing Gram stains of each isolate. Representative images were taken using the 1000X objective on a light microscope.

Bacterial sizes were highly varied between individual lactobacilli strains of the same species (**Figure 3.3A**). While there were no significant differences in bacterial sizes between the different species after adjusting for multiple comparisons, *L. ruminis* isolates tended to be the largest and *L. plantarum* isolates were the smallest (**Figure 3.3B**).

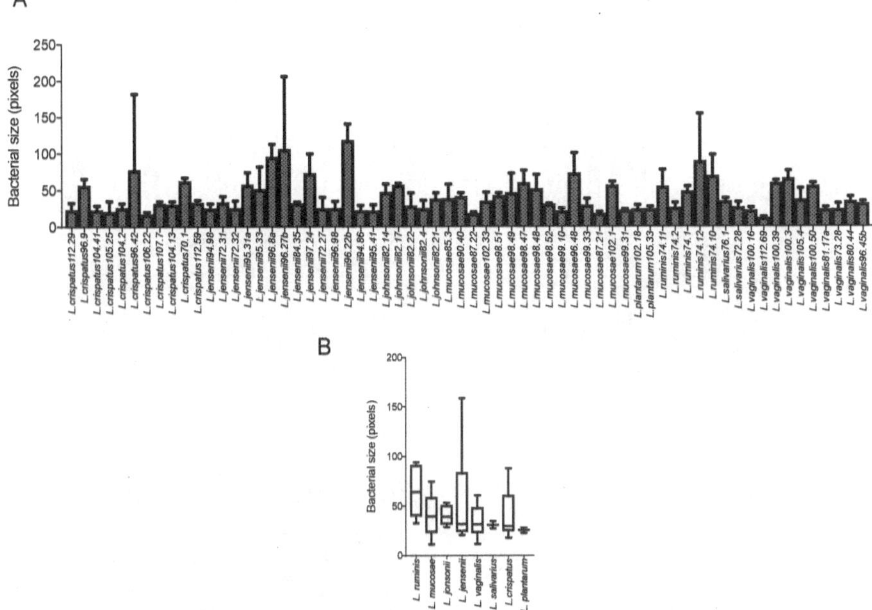

Figure 3.3: Sizes of vaginal *Lactobacillus* isolates. (**A**) Size of individual lactobacilli strains. Bars show the medians and ranges of five measurements for each isolate. (**B**) Sizes of *Lactobacillus* grouped by species. Data are shown as Tukey box plots. Boxes represent the interquartile ranges, lines within boxes represent medians and whiskers represent minimum and maximum values. Single colonies were picked from *Lactobacillus* cultures [including *L. crispatus* (n=11), *L. jensenii* (n=14), *L. johnsonii* (n=5), *L. mucosae* (n=15), *L. plantarum* (n=2), *L. ruminis* (n=5), *L. salivarius* (n=2), *L. vaginalis* (n=10)] and smears were prepared on microscope slides and Gram-stained before taking images at 1000X magnification. Bacterial size was determined from the images using Image J^{TM} software. Mann-Whitney U tests were used to compare bacterial sizes and p-values were adjusted for multiple comparisons using a false discovery rate step-down procedure. There were no significant differences between species after adjusting for multiple comparisons.

3.4.5 *Lactobacillus* growth rates and adhesion to vaginal epithelial cells

As bacterial adhesion to epithelial cells and growth rates are among the most important characteristics for colonisation and persistence of lactobacilli in the FGT (Gueimonde *et al.*, 2006; Osset *et al.*, 2002), these characteristics were assessed *in vitro.* All of the lactobacilli analysed were able to adhere to vaginal epithelial (VK2) cells, although the level of lactobacilli adhesion was highly varied, even between strains of the same species (**Figure 3.4A**) as well as between species

(**Figure 3.4B-C** and **Appendix III**). Although no statistically significant differences were observed between species, *L. ruminis* isolates had the lowest adhesion scores compared to the other isolates and *L. jensenii* were most adherent.

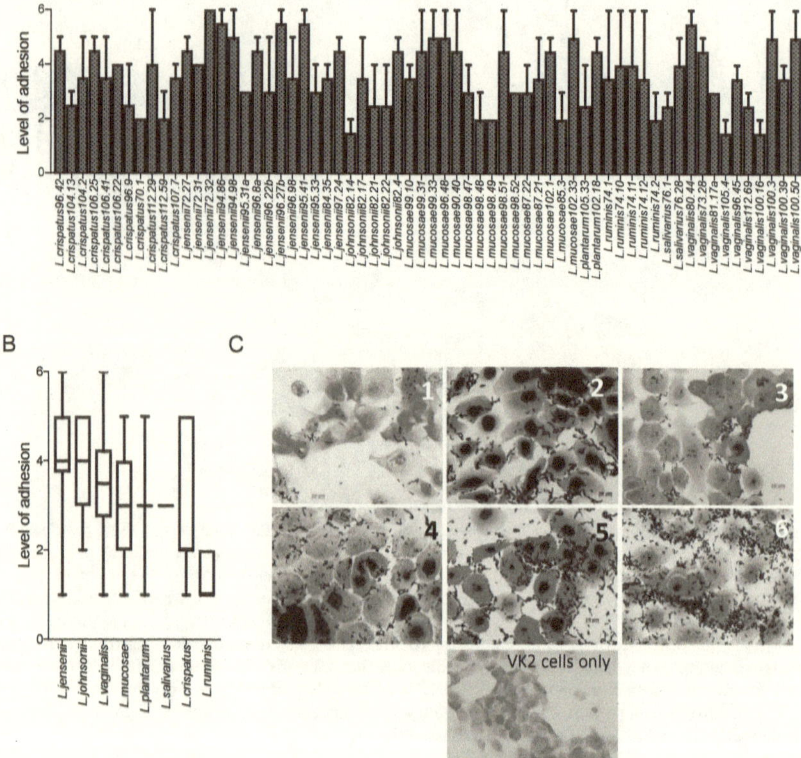

Figure 3.4: *Lactobacillus* adhesion to vaginal epithelial (VK2) cells. (A) Lactobacilli adhesion scores for individual lactobacilli isolates including [*L. crispatus* (n=11), *L. jensenii* (n=14), *L. johnsonii* (n=5), *L. mucosae* (n=15), *L. plantarum* (n=2), *L. ruminis* (n=5), *L. salivarius* (n=2), *L. vaginalis* (n=10)]. (**B**) Lactobacilli adhesion by species. Data are shown as Tukey box plots. Boxes represent the interquartile ranges, lines within boxes represent medians and whiskers represent minimum and maximum values. (**C**) Gram stained images showing *Lactobacillus* adhesion to VK2 cells. *Lactobacillus* isolates were cultured and adjusted to 4.18×10^6 colony forming units (CFU)/ml in antibiotic free keratinocyte serum free media before being added to VK2 cell monolayers in chamber slides and incubated for 2 hours at 37°C with 5% CO_2. Slides were then washed to remove unbound lactobacilli and Gram stained. Representative images of the Gram stained slides were collected and *Lactobacillus* isolates were ranked according to level of adhesion in ascending order from least adherent (**1**) to the most adherent (**6**).

Lactobacilli growth rates under anaerobic conditions were determined by measuring the OD_{600} of bacterial suspensions at six different time points from baseline up to 24 hours. The growth rates were also highly varied between individual strains of the same species and between different species (**Figure 3.5A**). However, *L. salivarius* isolates grew the fastest while *L. mucosae* isolates grew the slowest in MRS broth (**Figure 3.5B**).

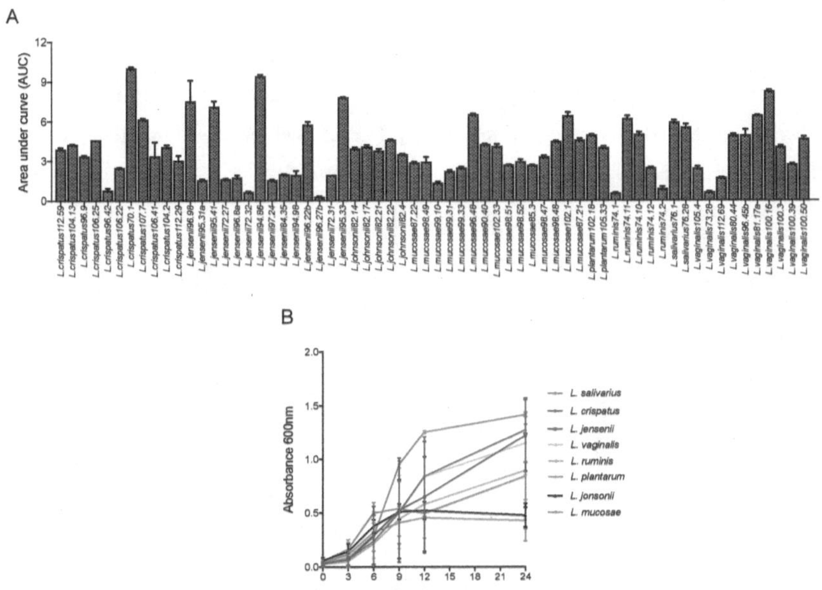

Figure 3.5: Lactobacilli growth rates. Lactobacilli isolates including [*L. crispatus* (n=11), *L. jensenii* (n=14), *L. johnsonii* (n=5), *L. mucosae* (n=15), *L. plantarum* (n=2), *L. ruminis* (n=5), *L. salivarius* (n=2), *L. vaginalis* (n=10)] were cultured and adjusted to 4.18×10^6 colony forming units (CFU)/ml, inoculated into 96-well plates in triplicate, before incubating anaerobically and measuring the optical density (OD_{600nm}) at six time points 3 hours apart from baseline up to 24 hours. (**A**) The bars represent the area under the curve (AUC) for each isolate that were determined during the active phase of growth (between 0 hours and 24 hours). (**B**) Growth curves of *Lactobacillus* isolates grouped by species.

Growth rates were not associated with bacterial size (Spearman rho=0.0068; p=0.9576), and there was no correlation between lactobacilli adhesion to VK2 cells and size (Spearman rho=-0.1182; p=0.3522) or growth rates (Spearman rho=-0.028; p=0.8243).

3.4.6 Lactic acid production and pH modification by *Lactobacillus* isolates

All of the lactobacilli isolates produced detectable amounts of D-lactate. *L. jensenii* isolates produced the most D-lactate while *L. salivarius* isolates produced the least (**Figure 3.6A**). L-lactate production was highly varied among the different species (**Figure 3.6B**) and there was no correlation between D and L-lactate production (Spearman rho= 0.0769; p= 0.5459). *L. johnsonii* isolates produced the largest amount of total lactic acid (**Figure 3.6C**), calculated using the Henderson-Hasselbach equation (O'Hanlon *et al.*, 2013). Culture pH values during the exponential phase of growth (24 hours) ranged from 3.78 to 5.6 and *L. salivarius* isolates acidified the culture medium the most, despite producing very little D- and L-lactate relative to the other species. Neither D- nor L-lactate correlated with culture pH while total lactic acid negatively correlated with culture pH (Spearman rho=0.9034; p<0.0001) (**Figure 3.7**).

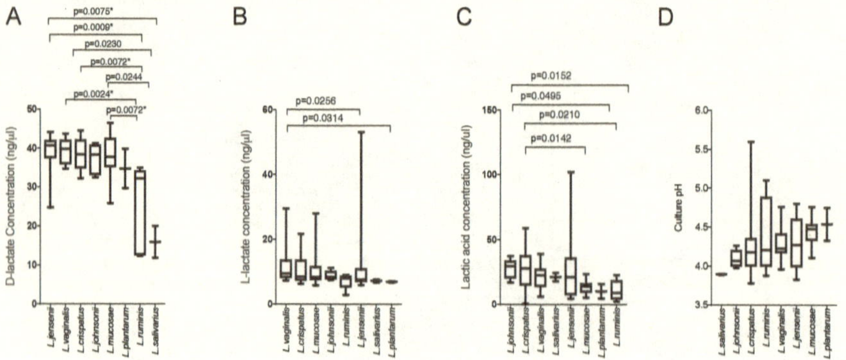

Figure 3.6: Comparison of (A) D-lactate production, (B) L-lactate production, (C) total lactic acid production and (D) culture acidification by clinical *Lactobacillus* isolates in culture. *Lactobacillus* isolates [*L. crispatus* (n=10), *L. jensenii* (n=14), *L. johnsonii* (n=5), *L. mucosae* (n=15), *L. plantarum* (n=2), *L. ruminis* (n=5), *L. salivarius* (n=2), *L. vaginalis* (n=10)] were cultured and adjusted to $4.18 x 10^6$ colony forming units (CFU)/ml in de Man Rogosa and Sharpe (MRS) broth then incubated anaerobically for 24 hours at 37°C. Supernatants were collected and the concentrations of D-lactate and L-lactate were determined by ELISA assays. Culture pH was measured using a pH meter. Total lactic acid was calculated using the Henderson-Hasselbach equation. Boxes represent the interquartile ranges, lines within boxes represent medians and whiskers represent minimum and maximum values. Mann-Whitney U tests were used to compare characteristics between *Lactobacillus* species and p-values were adjusted for multiple comparisons using a false discovery rate step down procedure. P-values <0.05 were considered statistically significant. *p values that remained significant after adjustment for multiple comparisons.

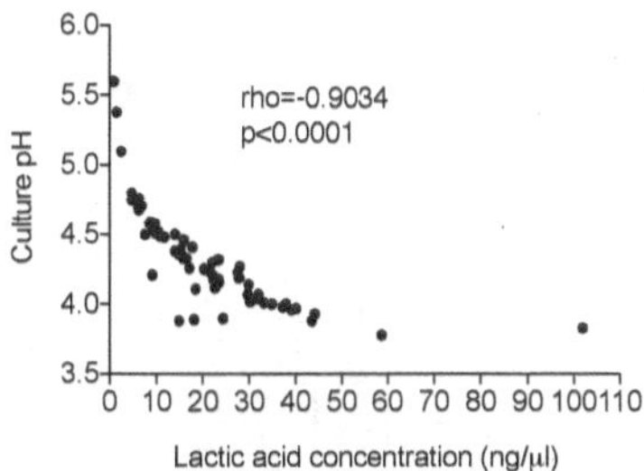

Figure 3.7: Correlation between culture pH and total lactic acid concentration produced by *Lactobacillus* isolates. *Lactobacillus* isolates (n=64) were cultured in de Man Rogosa and Sharpe (MRS) broth, adjusted to 4.18×10^6 colony forming units (CFU)/ml in MRS broth and incubated anaerobically for 24 hours at 37°C. Supernatants were collected and the concentrations of D-lactate and L-lactate were determined by ELISA assays. Culture pH was measured using a pH meter. Total lactic acid, calculated using the Henderson-Hasselbach equation, correlated with culture pH (Spearman rho=-0.9034, p<0.0001).

3.4.7 Evaluation of the relationships between participant characteristics and the properties of *Lactobacillus* isolates

To determine whether the vaginal environment from which the bacteria were isolated influenced the properties of lactobacilli, characteristics including level of adhesion to VK2 cells, growth rates, bacterial sizes, D- and L-lactate and lactic acid production and culture acidification were compared between isolates obtained from women with optimal microbiota and women with non-optimal microbiota (intermediate microbiota and BV). There were no significant differences in the levels of adhesion, growth rates and bacterial sizes among isolates obtained from women with optimal microbiota, intermediate microbiota and those obtained from women with non-optimal microbiota, suggesting that these characteristics are not associated with the development of BV (**Figure 3.8A-C**).

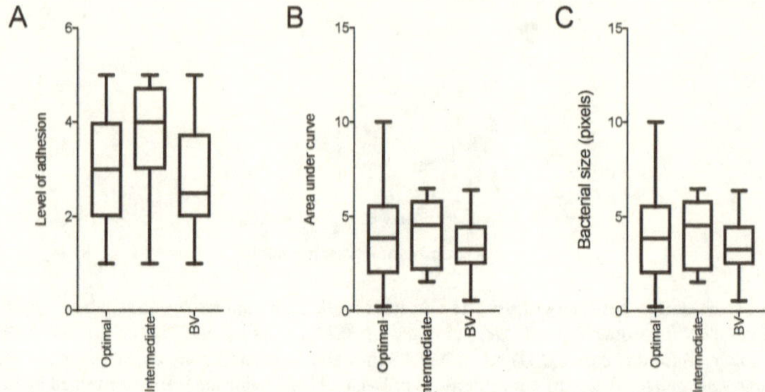

Figure 3.8: Level of adhesion to VK2 cells, growth rates and bacterial sizes of *Lactobacillus* isolates from women stratified by bacterial vaginosis (BV) status. *Lactobacillus* isolates were obtained from women with optimal (n=36), intermediate microbiota (n=8) and bacterial vaginosis (BV; n=20). (**A**) Adhesion was determined by adding *Lactobacillus* cultures adjusted to 4.18×10^6 colony forming units (CFU)/ml to VK2 cell monolayers and incubating for 2 hours at 37°C with 5% CO_2. Non-adherent bacteria were washed off with sterile phosphate buffered saline (PBS) before the slides were Gram-stained and the levels of adhesion scored. (**B**) Growth rates were evaluated by measuring the optical densities at a wavelength of 600nm, of *Lactobacillus* cultures initially adjusted to 4.18×10^6 CFU/ml, over time. The area under the curve (AUC) was calculated for each isolate during the active phase of growth (between 0 hours and 12 hours). (**C**) Bacterial size was determined by picking single colonies from *Lactobacillus* cultures, preparing smears on microscope slides and Gram-staining before taking images at 1000X magnification. Bacterial size was determined from the images using Image J™ software. Boxes represent the interquartile ranges, lines within boxes represent medians and whiskers represent minimum and maximum values. P-values <0.05 were considered statistically significant.

Lactobacilli isolates obtained from women with optimal microbiota produced significantly greater amounts of D-lactate compared with isolates from women with BV (p=0.0083) or intermediate microbiota (p=0.0194; **Figure 3.9A**). There were no significant differences in L-lactate production between isolates obtained from women with optimal, intermediate microbiota and BV (**Figure 3.9B**). Total lactic acid also differed significantly between the lactobacilli isolates from women with optimal microbiota versus BV (p=0.0457) (**Figure 3.9C**), while there were no differences observed in culture acidification (**Figure 3.9D**). Additionally, *L. jensenii* was isolated more frequently from women with optimal microbiota (p=0.0150), while *L. mucosae* (p=0.0156) and *L. ruminis* (p=0.0129) were more frequently isolated from women with non-optimal microbiota (**Figure 3.9E**). Overall, lactobacilli isolates from women with BV were less likely to produce D-lactate than those from women with optimal microbiota (adjusted OR: 0.84; 95% CI: 0.73-0.950; p=0.006) after adjusting for species.

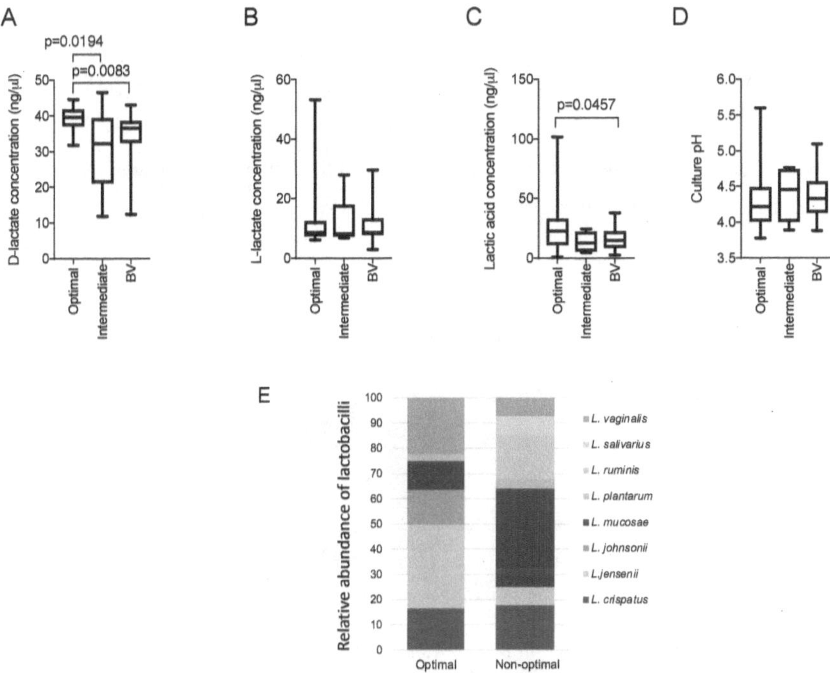

Figure 3.9: Comparison of (A) D-lactate production, (B) L-lactate production, (C) total lactic acid production and (D) culture acidification by clinical *Lactobacillus* isolates in bacterial culture and (E) relative abundance of *Lactobacillus* isolates from women stratified by bacterial vaginosis (BV) status. (**A-D**) *Lactobacillus* isolates, obtained from women with optimal (n=36) and non-optimal [bacterial vaginosis (n=20) and intermediate microbiota (n=8)], were cultured and adjusted to 4.18×10^6 colony forming units (CFU)/ml in de Man Rogosa and Sharpe (MRS) broth then incubated for 24 hours at 37°C. Supernatants were collected and the concentrations of D-lactate, L-lactate were determined by ELISA assays. Culture pH was measured using a pH meter in bacterial cultures. Total lactic acid was calculated using the Henderson-Hasselbach equation. Boxes represent the interquartile ranges, lines within boxes represent medians and whiskers represent minimum and maximum values. Mann-Whitney U tests were used to compare characteristics and $p<0.05$ was considered statistically significant. (**E**) Relative abundance of the lactobacilli species was expressed as percentage of the total number of isolates obtained from women with optimal [Nugent 0-3, (n=36)] and women with non-optimal microbiota [Nugent 4-10, (n=28)] in the respective group with the colours representing different species on the stacked bars. Fisher's exact test was used to compare the species between the two groups. P-values <0.05 were considered statistically significant.

As semen also contains *Lactobacillus* species and may be a source of isolates (Weng *et al.*, 2014), the relationships between the detection of PSA (an indicator of recent exposure to semen) and *Lactobacillus* properties were evaluated. Bacterial size was associated with semen contamination, with lactobacilli obtained from women with recent exposure to semen being smaller in size compared to isolates obtained from women with no semen contamination in their vaginal fluid (p=0.0025) (**Figure 3.10A**). Interestingly, *L. mucosae* was isolated more frequently from women who had recent unprotected sex (p=0.014; **Figure 3.10B**). Thus, semen contamination in the cervicovaginal fluid may have influenced the size or species of the lactobacilli present in the FGT or this could be a spurious association.

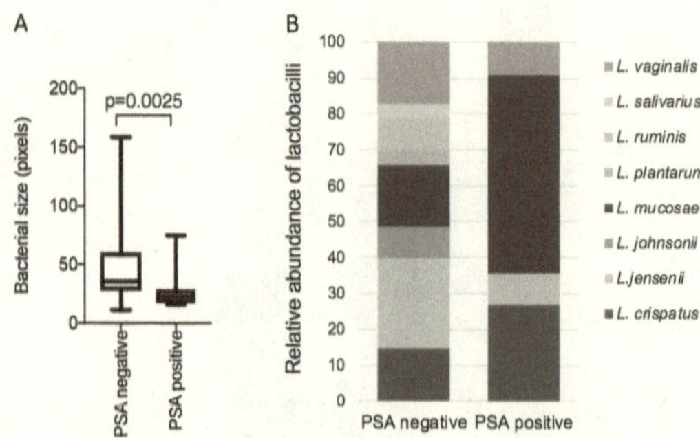

Figure 3.10: Sizes and species of *Lactobacillus* isolates from women with or without semen contamination in their mucosal secretions. (A) Single colonies were picked from *Lactobacillus* cultures, smears were prepared on microscope slides and Gram-stained before taking images at 1000x magnification. Bacterial size was determined from the images using Image J^{TM} software and compared between isolates obtained from women with no semen contamination (n=53) and women with contamination (n=11), determined by prostate specific antigen (PSA) ELISA. Data are shown as Tukey box plots. Boxes represent the interquartile ranges, lines within boxes represent medians and whiskers represent minimum and maximum values. Mann-Whitney U tests were used to compare bacterial sizes and $p<0.05$ was considered statistically significant. (**B**) Lactobacilli species isolated from women with and without semen contamination. The colours represent different species on the stacked bars as percentages of the total number of lactobacilli in the respective group.

Lactobacillus isolates obtained from women with STI infections produced more lactic acid (p=0.0246) and acidified culture medium better (p=0.0374) than isolates from women without STI infections (**Figure 3.11A**). Additionally, *L. mucosae* (p=0.0482) isolates were more common in women who had no STI infections while *L. johnsonii* (p=0.0011) isolates were more common in women with STI infections (**Figure 3.11C**). However, there was no association between the presence of an STI and bacterial size or lactobacilli adhesion to vaginal epithelial cells. Following adjustment for BV status, the presence of STIs did not remain significantly associated with total lactic acid.

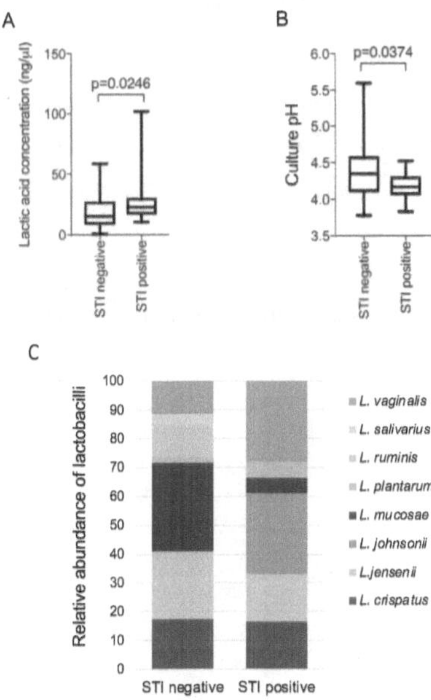

Figure 3.11: Lactic acid production, culture acidification and relative abundance of *Lactobacillus* isolates from women stratified by sexually transmitted infections (STI) status. (A) *Lactobacillus* isolates, obtained from women who had no STI (n=46) and women who were STI positive (n=18), were cultured and adjusted to 4.18×10^6 colony forming units (CFU)/ml in de Man Rogosa and Sharpe (MRS) broth then incubated for 24 hours at 37°C. Supernatants were collected and the concentrations of D-lactate, L-lactate were determined by ELISA assays and total lactic acid was calculated using the Henderson-Hasselbach equation. (**B**) Culture pH was measured using a pH meter in bacterial cultures. Boxes represent the interquartile ranges, lines within boxes represent medians and whiskers represent minimum and maximum values. (**C**) Relative abundance of the lactobacilli species was expressed as percentage of the total number of isolates in the respective group with the colours representing different species on the stacked bars. Fisher's exact test was used to compare the species between the two groups. P-values <0.05 were considered statistically significant.

3.4.8 Overall performance of *Lactobacillus* isolates

A scoring system was formulated in order to compare and rank the lactobacilli based on the characteristics analysed in this Chapter. Each isolate was given a score per characteristic analysed, including (1) level of adhesion to epithelial cells; the levels of (2) D-, (3) L-lactate produced, (4) growth rates and (5) culture acidification (pH) (**Table 3.2**). Relative scores per category, except pH, were assigned as follows: <25th percentile (score = 0); 25th–50th percentile (score = 1); 50th-75th percentile score (score = 2); ≥75th (score = 3). Isolates that acidified the culture medium the most were scored higher, so the scores were as follows: *Lactobacillus* strains with culture pH between 3.5-4 scored 3 points, 4-4.5 scored 2 points, 4.5-5 scored 1 point and more than 5 scored 0 points.

Table 3.2 Phenotypic characteristics of vaginal lactobacilli isolates

Species	Adhesion	Growth rates	Size	D-lactate	L-lactate	Culture pH	Total score
L.vaginalis	6	2	3	1	3	2	17
L.mucosae	4	3	3	2	3	2	17
L.mucosae	6	3	2	1	3	2	17
L.jensenii	4	0	2	3	3	4	16
L.vaginalis	6	2	2	2	2	2	16
L.johnsonii	5	2	2	3	1	3	16
L.jensenii	5	0	3	2	3	3	16
L.johnsonii	6	2	1	1	2	3	15
L.vaginalis	6	1	3	2	2	1	15
L.vaginalis	3	3	1	3	3	2	15
L.crispatus	3	3	1	3	3	2	15
L.jensenii	6	3	2	3	0	1	15
L.vaginalis	4	3	0	3	3	2	15
L.crispatus	6	1	1	1	3	3	15
L.mucosae	3	2	2	3	3	2	15
L.jensenii	4	0	1	3	3	3	14
L.johnsonii	3	2	3	2	1	3	14
L.jensenii	6	3	0	2	0	3	14
L.jensenii	4	0	2	3	3	2	14
L.jensenii	6	0	3	3	0	2	14
L.crispatus	4	1	3	3	0	3	14
L.mucosae	6	2	3	1	1	1	14
L.crispatus	6	2	0	1	3	2	14
L.salivarius	6	3	1	0	1	3	14
L.johnsonii	4	2	2	1	2	2	13
L.johnsonii	4	2	1	2	2	2	13
L.crispatus	5	0	3	3	2	0	13
L.vaginalis	5	2	2	1	2	1	13
L.crispatus	4	3	3	3	0	0	13
L.mucosae	3	1	2	3	3	1	13
L.crispatus	3	1	1	2	3	3	13

Species	**Adhesion**	**Growth rates**	**Bacterial size**	**D-lactate**	**L-lactate**	**Culture pH**	**Total score**
L.mucosae	6	**2**	**0**	**1**	**2**	**2**	**13**
L.jensenii	5	0	1	3	0	3	12
L.mucosae	6	1	1	1	2	1	12
L.vaginalis	2	3	0	3	1	3	12
L.jensenii	2	3	3	1	2	1	12
L.jensenii	4	3	0	2	0	3	12
L.ruminis	2	3	3	1	1	2	12
L.salivarius	4	3	2	0	0	3	12
L.jensenii	6	0	0	1	2	2	11
L.vaginalis	1	1	2	3	2	2	11
L.ruminis	2	3	3	0	0	3	11
L.mucosae	2	1	3	2	2	1	11
L.mucosae	3	1	2	2	1	2	11
L.crispatus	3	2	1	1	2	2	11
L.jensenii	4	0	3	2	1	1	11
L.mucosae	5	0	0	1	2	2	10
L.plantarum	4	2	0	2	0	2	10
L.crispatus	2	1	1	2	1	3	10
L.vaginalis	4	0	0	1	3	2	10
L.crispatus	1	2	1	3	0	3	10
L.mucosae	4	2	2	0	0	2	10
L.mucosae	2	1	3	1	2	1	10
L.mucosae	3	1	0	2	2	2	10
L.vaginalis	5	0	0	3	1	1	10
L.plantarum	6	2	1	0	0	1	10
L.crispatus	2	1	0	2	2	2	9
L.jensenii	6	0	1	0	1	1	9
L.jensenii	2	3	0	2	0	1	8
L.ruminis	1	1	3	0	1	2	8
L.mucosae	4	0	0	1	1	1	7
L.ruminis	1	0	2	1	2	1	7

Species	Adhesion	Growth rates	Bacterial size	D-lactate	L-lactate	Culture pH	Total score
L.ruminis	1	0	1	1	2	0	5
L.mucosae	1	1	0	1	1	1	5

3.5 Discussion

Identification and evaluation of the differences in characteristics between *Lactobacillus* species and strains present in the FGT may explain the differences in susceptibility of women to recurrent BV, as well as STIs. Previous studies have described variation among *Lactobacillus* strains regarding adherence to the FGT epithelium, competitive inhibition of pathogen adherence to the epithelium and growth inhibition (Osset *et al*., 2001; Sanders *et al*., 2008; Verstraelen *et al*., 2009). Among the properties thought to be beneficial to the host and important for colonization and persistence are lactic acid and H_2O_2 production (O'Hanlon *et al*., 2011; Gong *et al*., 2014; Hearps *et al*., 2017; Tyssen *et al*., 2018), bacteriocin production, viability, bacterial size and adhesion to epithelial cells (Boris *et al*., 1998; Osset *et al*., 2002; Gueimonde *et al*., 2006; Gueimonde & Salminen, 2006; Borgdorff *et al*., 2014; Breshears *et al*., 2015; Matsubara *et al*., 2016). In this Chapter, *in vitro* growth rates, bacterial sizes, adhesion to vaginal epithelial cells, lactate production and culture acidification were compared among 64 vaginal lactobacilli isolated from South African women. When the species were scored according to the various characteristics evaluated including adhesion, growth rates, sizes, D-lactate and L-lactate production and culture acidification, there was substantial variation within each species, with some strains performing well and others performing relatively poorly. Therefore, there was no particular species as a group that could be named as the best performing group. However, when compared among the top ten strains, *L. crispatus* and *L. jensenii* isolates were the most common isolates. Total lactic acid and D-lactate production differed significantly between isolates obtained from women with optimal microbiota and those obtained from women with non-optimal microbiota. *L. jensenii* species was more frequently isolated in women with optimal microbiota. Additionally, the presence of an STI or semen contamination was associated with the size or species of lactobacilli isolated from the women, with bacterial size inversely associated with semen contamination.

FGTs colonised by *L. crispatus* have been considered to have the most stable optimal vaginal microbiota in young women as this species has been associated with a decreased risk of inflammation and reduced risk of HIV acquisition (Doerflinger *et al*., 2014; Gosmann *et al*., 2017). Additionally, *L. crispatus* has also been associated with pH reduction in the FGT and reduced risk of conversion from optimal to non-optimal vaginal microbiota (Boskey *et al*., 1999; Pendharkar *et al*., 2013; Verstraelen *et al*., 2009). It has also been shown that *L. crispatus* inhibits the growth of *G. vaginalis* and *N. gonorrhoeae* on porcine vaginal mucosa (Breshears *et al*., 2015) and has better antagonistic activity against *E. coli* and *Candida* spp. compared to *L. gasseri* and *L. jensenii* (Breshears *et al*., 2015; Hütt *et al*., 2016). However, *L. crispatus* dominance is rare in African women, with the majority who have *Lactobacillus* dominance being colonised by *L. iners* (Anahtar *et al*., 2015; Lennard *et al*., 2017). Lower frequencies of *L. crispatus* and *L. jensenii* have also been observed in black and Hispanic women in comparison to white women and Asian women in the USA (Zhou *et al*., 2007; Pendharkar *et al*., 2013; Martínez-Peña *et al*., 2013; Williams *et al*., 2016; Hütt *et al*., 2016). The reasons for this are currently unknown, although genetic factors (Ravel *et al*., 2011), behavioural factors (hygiene, contraceptive use and sexual behavior; Schwebke *et al*., 2009; Ravel *et al*., 2011), as well as the properties of the microbiota present may play a role. It is thus essential to improve our understanding of optimal versus non-optimal vaginal microbiota in this population. Furthermore, the presence or dominance of lactobacilli in the FGT is critical for protection against uropathogens, which are highly prevalent in African women (Cherpes *et al*., 2003; Wiesenfeld *et al*., 2003; Brotman, 2011; Gillet *et al*., 2011; Rathod *et al*., 2012; Lennard *et al*., 2017; Eastment & McClelland, 2018; Osset *et al*., 2001; Borgdorff *et al*., 2014; Breshears *et al*., 2015). However, recent studies have shown that some of these women whose FGTs are colonised by lactobacilli still develop BV, suggesting differences in the capacity to protect between strains and/ or species (Sanders, 2008). In this Chapter, *L. mucosae* was most frequently isolated from the vaginal samples followed by *L. jensenii, L. crispatus* and *L. vaginalis. L. johnsonii, L. ruminis, L. salivarius* and *L. plantarum*. *L. crispatus* and *L. jensenii* isolates from this cohort of African women performed particularly well compared to other species when probiotic properties were assessed.

Lactobacilli adhesion to the epithelial mucosa is a critical step for successful colonization, contributing to the exclusion of pathogens as they compete for binding sites (Osset *et al*., 2001; Gueimonde *et al*., 2006; Homayouni *et al*., 2014; Santarmaki *et al*., 2017). Adhesion promotes persistence by placing the lactobacilli in close contact with epithelial cells and increasing retention time of the lactobacilli in the FGT (Gueimonde *et al*., 2006). Atassi *et al*. (2006) showed that lactobacilli inhibit adherence of *G. vaginalis* and *P. bivia* to HeLa cells. In the current Chapter, *L. jensenii* isolates were the most adherent, while *L. ruminis* isolates were the least adherent to vaginal epithelial cells. These differences were not however statistically significant and there was a large amount of variation within species, as well as between the species, as previously reported (Andreu *et al*., 1995; Osset *et al*., 2002). This suggests that adhesion is strain specific. It is not clear whether the level of *in vitro* adhesion observed here reflects the level of lactobacilli persistence *in vivo,* as successful adhesion is influenced by multiple factors, including the production of different surface proteins involved in adhesion, the presence of cervicovaginal mucus and vaginal pH (Alander *et al*., 1999; Zoetendal *et al*., 2002; Borgdorff *et al*., 2015). Further studies would need to be carried out in order to assess whether *in vitro* adhesion is fully indicative of persistence in the FGT, as well as tolerance to conditions in the FGT (Osset *et al*., 2001).

In this Chapter, there was a large amount of variation in growth rates between strains of the same species and between species. Although growth rates were evaluated *in vitro* in the current study, it is also not clear whether these results correspond with what actually takes place *in vivo.* A previous review suggested that measuring the production of metabolites produced by lactobacilli such as lactic acid might be linked to growth and viability (Gueimonde & Salminen, 2006). However, neither D nor L-lactate production correlated with the growth rates of the lactobacilli analysed in this Chapter. Larger bacterial size and rapid bacterial multiplication have been associated with improved capability to adhere to epithelial cells (Mastromarino *et al*., 2002), but contrary to past reports, bacterial size and growth rates were not correlated with adhesion in this study.

All isolates produced D-lactate, while only some produced L-lactate and there was a large amount of variation in these properties between strains, even within species. Additionally, isolates from women with non-optimal microbiota produced significantly lower amounts of D-lactate and lactic acid. This suggests that the amount of vaginal lactic acid is largely dependent on the particular *Lactobacillus* species or strains that predominate, as previously suggested (Witkin *et al*., 2013). Additionally, as lactic acid contributes to maintaining a pH below 4.5 in the FGT which hinders the growth of BV-associated bacteria and pathogens (Aldunate *et al*., 2013; O'Hanlon *et al*., 2013), the lower amounts of lactic acid produced by isolates from women with non-optimal microbiota may reflect their inability to protect against colonization by non-optimal bacteria.

Interestingly, there were no significant differences in the levels of adhesion, bacterial sizes and growth rates between isolates obtained from women with optimal versus non-optimal microbiota and therefore, it is not clear whether differences in these properties evaluated are influential in the conversion from an optimal to a non-optimal vaginal microbiome. However, *Lactobacillus* isolates obtained from women with optimal microbiota produced more D-lactate and total lactic acid than those of women with intermediate microbiota and BV. The finding that three of the lactobacilli species were differentially abundant between women with non-optimal versus optimal microbiota may be due to varying production of metabolites, such as lactic acid in this case.

It has been shown in the past that the microorganisms described on labels do not always correspond with what is contained in the probiotic formulations (Temmerman *et al.*, 2003; Happel *et al.*, 2017). Species level identification is thus critical. Here, MALDI-TOF biotyping was used to identify isolated bacteria to species level. An alternative method, 16s rRNA sequencing, often fails to differentiate between species that are closely related such as *L. casei* and *L. paracasei* or *L. pentosus* and *L. plantarum*, due to similarities in certain variable regions of the 16S rRNA gene sequences that are amplified (Anderson *et al.*, 2014; Huang *et al.*, 2014). In addition, 16S rRNA gene sequencing is time and labour-consuming, relatively expensive and unsuitable for routine identification (Duskova *et al.*, 2012). On the other hand, MALDI-TOF has been described as a simple, cost effective and reliable rapid method suitable for the characterisation of lactobacilli which allows pooling of samples in one analysis (Anderson *et al.*, 2014; Dec *et al.*, 2016; Dec *et al.*, 2014; Kern *et al.*, 2014; Sato *et al.*, 2012; Zhang *et al.*, 2014). However, MALDI-TOF requires that bacterial colonies are less than 48 hours old as colonies cultivated for a longer period may result in weaker and less distinguished peaks in the spectra. In this book, MALDI-TOF biotyping was thus performed on fresh lactobacilli colonies. Although typing by polymerase chain reaction (PCR) is much more time consuming than MALDI-TOF due to the requirement for DNA extraction, PCR amplification and electrophoresis, identification based on DNA analysis has been described as the most reliable method and has greater precision due to the possibility of typing strains at the intraspecies level (Dec *et al.*, 2014).

A limitation of this study was that all the assays were carried out *in vitro* and the observations made may not necessarily correspond with *in vivo* conditions. In addition to this limitation, for some of the strains analysed here, very few isolates were obtained and this limited the statistical power for the respective species. It is also worth noting that *L. iners* was not isolated from any of the participants as selective media for this species was not included in the study protocol. Additionally, the aim of this book was to evaluate the antimicrobial properties of vaginal *Lactobacillus* species that are considered to be optimal in the female genital tract and associated with minimal or low levels of inflammatory cytokines in the female genital tract to identify isolates that may potentially be used to improve the current probiotics formulations. The role of *L. iners* is controversial since this species has been associated with increased risk of conversion from an optimal to a non-optimal vaginal microbiome in women (Verstraelen *et al.*, 2009). Therefore, *L. iners* was excluded from the characterisation. Further studies including *L. iners* may be important to investigate differences in the characteristics evaluated in this Chapter between *L. iners* and other *Lactobacillus* species.

In conclusion, the findings in this Chapter suggest that the protective lactobacilli characteristics considered important for vaginal re-colonization are strain specific, as previously described in isolates obtained from European women (Atassi *et al.*, 2006) and that the vaginal environment may have an influence on the lactobacilli properties. These findings highlight the importance of thoroughly screening large numbers of species and strains obtained from different women to identify the best performing strains for probiotic development as there seems to be a large amount of variation in protective characteristics. Furthermore, this highlights the diversity of microbial function that likely plays a critical role in health and disease, but is not evaluated using measures of abundance such as 16S rRNA amplicon sequencing.

CHAPTER 4: Comparison of antimicrobial characteristics between commercial probiotics and vaginal *Lactobacillus* isolates from young South African women

4.1 Summary

BV is associated with an upregulation of inflammatory cytokines in the FGT increasing the risk of HIV acquisition and STIs. Probiotics have shown potential to improve BV treatment outcomes and restore the normal vaginal microbiota, however substantial heterogeneity in efficacy has been observed during clinical trials. Additionally, there are only a few vaginal probiotics available commercially and most contain strains that are not normally found in the FGT. In this Chapter, probiotic-relevant characteristics were compared between commercially available vaginal probiotics and vaginal *Lactobacillus* isolates in order to evaluate the potential to improve existing probiotic formulations. The antimicrobial (culture acidification, size, growth rates, adhesion, D-lactate and L-lactate production) characteristics of 23 vaginal *Lactobacillus* isolates from South African women, two commercial probiotics, Provacare (containing *L. casei rhamnosus*) and Vagiforte (which is supplied as vaginal pessaries and oral capsules that contain *L. acidophilus*) and 4 reference strains were evaluated. Interestingly, the vaginal lactobacilli generally performed better than the probiotics according to the criteria used in this Chapter. The findings suggest that there is significant potential for developing an improved vaginal probiotic using *Lactobacillus* strains isolated from healthy women for adjunctive therapy for BV. *L. jensenii* isolates may have the most potential as vaginal probiotics as these isolates were the most adherent, suggesting the potential for persistence in the genital tract and produced the most antimicrobial L-lactate.

4.2 Introduction

BV remains highly prevalent worldwide, largely because current treatment strategies are only partially effective (Bradshaw *et al.*, 2006; Cauci, 2004; McLean *et al.*, 2000). BV is characterised by changes in the normal vaginal microbiota in which the normally predominant *Lactobacillus* species have been replaced by diverse non-*Lactobacillus* communities (Fredricks *et al.*, 2005; Srinivasan *et al.*, 2008; Ravel *et al.*, 2011). The current standard-of-care for BV involves administration of oral or gel metronidazole and/or intravaginal clindamycin (Bradshaw *et al.*, 2006). Approximately 60-80% of women with BV are cured after antibiotic treatment (Hay, 2009). However, high recurrence rates have been reported of up to 40% of women within 3 months after antibiotic therapy and up to 50% of women after 6 months (Bradshaw *et al.*, 2006; Hay, 2009). Other side effects that have been associated with antibiotic therapy include superinfections by bacterial pathogens (Sobel *et al.*, 2006; Mastromarino *et al.*, 2013), as well as lactobacilli susceptibility to antimicrobial agents (Danielsen *et al.*, 2003). Moreover, studies have also reported emergence of drug resistance in anaerobic vaginal pathogens such as *G. vaginalis* (Mclean *et al.*, 1996; Beigi *et al.*, 2004).

Since the current standard of care has been associated with high recurrence rates, a complementary strategy to antibiotic treatment is oral or vaginal probiotic administration to recolonize the FGT with optimal *Lactobacillus* species and restore the normal vaginal microbiota (Andreu *et al.*, 1995; Bradshaw *et al.*, 2006; Hemmerling *et al.*, 2010; Larsson *et al.*, 2008). Several clinical trials have been conducted to assess the efficacy of orally or intravaginally administered probiotics on their own or as complementary treatment after antibiotic therapy (Anukam *et al.*, 2006; Falagas *et al.*, 2007; Mastromarino *et al.*, 2009; Machado *et al.*, 2016; Eriksson *et al.*, 2005; Larsson *et al.*, 2008; Petricevic *et al.*, 2008; Bradshaw *et al.*, 2012; Hemalatha *et al.*, 2012; Ling *et al.*, 2013; Bisanz *et al.*, 2014; Verdenelli *et al.*, 2016; Bohbot *et al.*, 2018; Rapisarda *et al.*, 2018). The use of probiotics after antibiotic treatment has shown an increase in BV cure rate and reduced recurrence rates in some studies, although none of the trials reported colonisation beyond the treatment period (Anukam *et al.*, 2006; Petricevic *et al*, 2008; Larsson *et al.*, 2008; van de Wijgert *et al.*, 2019). Probiotics may also be administered along with prebiotics to specifically support the growth of probiotic bacteria and increase the likelihood of persistence (Collins *et al.*, 2018). It is, however, still not yet clear whether intravaginal or oral administration is the more effective route of administration and the optimal *Lactobacillus* species for effective vaginal colonization remains unknown .

Probiotics are described as live organisms which can exert therapeutic benefits when administered in sufficient amounts (WHO, 2002; Hill *et al.*, 2014). The ability of the lactobacilli to multiply in the FGT would ensure an increase in size of the probiotic population. This, in turn, may increase the concentrations of protective metabolites secreted, improving the beneficial effects (Gueimonde *et al.*, 2006). A study carried out in European women showed that administration of heat-inactivated probiotic lactobacilli was associated with adverse outcomes such as gastrointestinal symptoms and diarrhea highlighting the importance of viability, although this was demonstrated in the gastrointestinal tract (Kirjavainen *et al.*, 2003). The characteristics of effective probiotics also include lactic acid production and adherence to vaginal epithelial cells (Boris *et al.*, 1998; Boskey *et al.*, 2001). Adherence to vaginal epithelial cells is a crucial step for successful vaginal colonization (Gueimonde *et al.*, 2006). Lactobacilli are able to competitively exclude pathogens in the FGT through adhesion to epithelial cells, facilitated by formation of microcolonies that cover epithelial cell receptors, preventing pathogen binding (Osset *et al.*, 2001) while lactic acid creates an acidic environment that inhibits pathogens (O'Hanlon *et al.*, 2011; Aldunate *et al.*, 2013). The morphology of the lactobacilli has also been shown to play an important role, with the longer strains covering a greater epithelial surface area and therefore inhibiting adherence of BV-associated bacteria (McLean *et al.*, 2000).

Currently, there are only a few vaginal probiotics available commercially and most contain strains that are not normally found in the FGT (Hughes *et al.*, 1990; Happel *et al.*, 2017). Additionally, different *Lactobacillus* species may differ in their capacity to protect due to species or strain variability (Osset *et al.*, 2001; Sanders, 2008; Hans Verstraelen *et al.*, 2009). The most common *Lactobacillus* species associated with genital health include *L. crispatus*, *L. jensenii*, *L. johnsonii*, *L. gasseri*, *L. vaginalis*, *L. mucosae*, *L. acidophilus* *L. plantarum* and *L. salivarius* although differences in the composition of the vaginal microbiota have been reported in different ethnic groups and geographical locations (Anukam *et al.*, 2005; Fredricks *et al.*, 2005; Ravel *et al.*, 2011; Petrova *et al.*, 2013). Interestingly, vaginal bacterial communities that are not dominated by *Lactobacillus* species are common among asymptomatic black women and it is therefore not clear what is considered optimal in this population. *L. crispatus,* in particular, is more frequently isolated from Caucasian women than African women (Anahtar *et al.*, 2015; Klatt *et al.*, 2017; Lennard *et al.*, 2017; Ravel *et al.*, 2011).

Here, the probiotic relevant characteristics of the only two topical vaginal probiotics found on the South African market were analysed and compared to vaginal lactobacilli isolated from South African women. The hypothesis was that vaginal lactobacilli isolated from South African women will improve the existing probiotics.

4.3 Methods

The *Lactobacillus* isolates analysed in this Chapter include 23 lactobacilli isolated from cervicovaginal fluid by Dr Remy Froissart and Mrs Hoyam Gamieldien and stored as described in Chapter 2. The aim of this analysis was to compare the probiotic-relevant characteristics of clinical *Lactobacillus* isolates to existing vaginal probiotics. For these assays, it is important to conduct the analysis of each isolate within the same experiment. Thus, in order to avoid repeating the same characterisation experiments on the same isolates described in Chapter 3, a random selection of novel isolates together with the vaginal probiotics was included in this section. The isolates were identified to species level using MALDI-TOF biotyping as *L. crispatus* (n=7), *L. jensenii* (n=5), *L. gasseri* (n=1), *L. mucosae* (n=4) and *L. vaginalis* (n=6). Four American Type Culture Collection (ATCC) reference strains (*L. jensenii* ATCC 25258, *L. gasseri* ATCC 9857, *L. crispatus* ATCC 33197 and 33820) were included in this analysis. Two commercial probiotics, Provacare (containing *L. casei rhamnosus*) and Vagiforte (which is supplied as vaginal pessaries and oral capsules that contain *L. acidophilus* and *Bifidobacterium longum* species) were obtained from a local pharmacy and a health store in Cape Town, South Africa. The isolation of lactobacilli from the commercial probiotics is described in Chapter 2. Growth rates for each isolate were determined by measuring the OD of cultures over time, (Chapter 2, section 2.10). D- and L-lactate production by the lactobacilli were evaluated using ELISA. The level of *Lactobacillus* adhesion to cervicovaginal epithelial cells (Ca Ski) was determined by incubating the isolates with Ca Ski cell monolayers for 2 hours. The cells were then washed three times with PBS to remove unbound bacteria, Gram-stained and images were collected for scoring of the levels of adhesion. Dr Emily Chetwin measured culture pH changes using a pH meter and conducted some of the adhesion analysis. The properties were then compared between commercial probiotics, vaginal *Lactobacillus* isolates and ATCC reference strains. The *Bifidobacterium* species were not isolated for the purposes of this dissertation.

4.4 Results

4.4.1 Study population

The vaginal *Lactobacillus* isolates analysed in this Chapter were obtained from 20 women aged between 16-22 years who participated in the WISH study in Cape Town (Barnabas *et al.*, 2018). All of the women were using hormonal contraceptives at the time of sample collection. Two women were BV positive, one woman had a *C. trachomatis* infection and six did not have an STI. All of the women were PCR negative for HSV-1, HSV-2, *M. genitalium*, *N. gonorrhoeae*, *T. pallidum* and *T. vaginalis* (**Table 4.1**).

Table 4.1: Demographic and clinical characteristics of study participants.

Demographic characteristics	**n (%)**
Black race	9 (100)
Median age in years (range)	18 (17-21)
Clinical and laboratory findings	**n (%)**
No STI or bacterial vaginosis	6 (66.7)
Bacterial vaginosis (Nugent ≥ 7)	2 (22.2)
Intermediate microbiota (Nugent 4-6)	0 (0)
Chlamydia trachomatis (PCR positive)	1 (11.1)
Neisseria gonorrhea (PCR positive)	0 (0)
Trichomonas vaginalis (PCR positive)	0 (0)
Mycoplasma genitalium (PCR positive)	0 (0)
HSV-2 IgG	0 (0)
HSV (PCR positive)	0 (0)
Treponema pallidum (RPR>1:4,TPHA positive)	0 (0)
Yeast cells	1 (11.1)
Contraception	
*Petogen	2 (22.2)
*Nur-Isterate	7 (77.8)

STI, sexually transmitted infection; PCR, polymerase chain reaction; HSV-2, herpes simplex virus type 2; RPR, rapid plasma reagin; TPHA, Treponema pallidum hemagglutination. *Progesterone-based injectables.

4.4.2 *Lactobacillus* isolation, size and growth rates

Twenty-three vaginal *Lactobacillus* isolates obtained from the women were identified to species level as *L. crispatus* (n=7), *L. gasseri* (n=1), *L. jensenii* (n=5), *L. mucosae* (n=4) and *L. vaginalis* (n=6). Two commercial probiotics were also included and the species from these were confirmed as *L. acidophilus* in the vaginal tablet and oral formulation (VagiForte), and *L. casei rhamnosus* (Provacare) in a capsule. Four ATCC reference strains (*L. crispatus* ATCC 33197), *L. crispatus* ATCC 33820, *L. gasseri* ATCC 9857, *L. jensenii* ATCC 25258) were also included. The numbers of viable bacteria present in cultures with an OD of 0.1$\pm$0.01 were determined and the CFU/ml calculated for each isolate (described in Chapter 2, section 2.7). This allowed for the standardisation of each culture prior to each experiment using spectrophotometry. **Figure 4.1A** shows the CFU/ml of cultures standardized to OD_{600} 0.1$\pm$0.01. There was marked variation in bacterial sizes (measured by Dr Emily Chetwin) and growth rates between individual strains of the same species and between different species (**Figure 4.1B-E**). The *L. casei rhamnosus* probiotic grew most rapidly, followed by the *L. crispatus* isolates and the *L. acidophilus* probiotic (**Figure 4.1D**), although the differences observed were not statistically significant. All of the lactobacilli isolated were viable in culture.

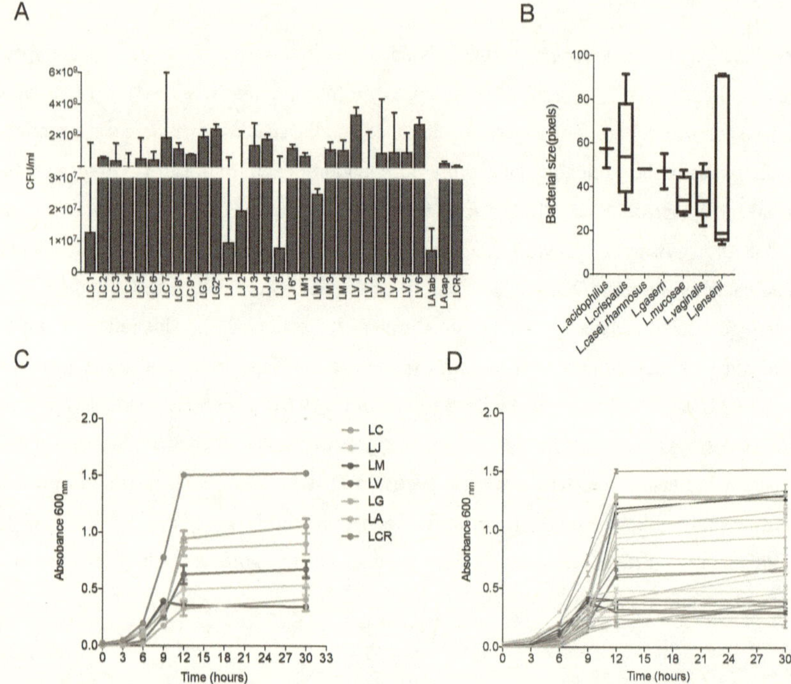

Figure 4.1: Number of colony forming units (CFU)/ml in standardized cultures, sizes and growth rates of lactobacilli isolates. (**A**) Lactobacilli were cultured in de Man Rogosa and Sharpe (MRS) broth, adjusted to an optical density at 600nm (OD_{600}) of 0.1±0.01, serially diluted and then plated on MRS agar plates in triplicate. After incubation for 24 hours under anaerobic conditions, CFUs were manually counted and CFU/ml for cultures standardized to OD_{600} 0.1±0.01 calculated for each isolate. Data are presented as medians and ranges. (**B**) Average bacterial sizes for *Lactobacillus* species. Single colonies were picked from *Lactobacillus* cultures, smears were prepared on microscope slides and Gram-stained before taking images at 1000X magnification. Bacterial size was determined from the images using Image J™ software. Data are shown as Tukey box plots. Boxes represent the interquartile ranges, lines within boxes represent medians and whiskers represent minimum and maximum values. Mann-Whitney U tests were used to compare bacterial sizes and p-values were adjusted for multiple comparisons using a false discovery rate step down procedure. No statistically significant differences (adjusted $p<0.05$) were noted. (**C-D**) *Lactobacillus* growth rates by species and by isolate are shown with symbols indicating means and error bars indicating the standard errors of the means of different isolates of the same species. LC, *Lactobacillus crispatus*; LG, *Lactobacillus gasseri*; LJ, *Lactobacillus jensenii*; LM, *Lactobacillus mucosae*; LV, *Lactobacillus vaginalis*. *LC 8, *Lactobacillus crispatus* ATCC 33197; *LC 9, *Lactobacillus crispatus* ATCC 33820; *LG 2, *Lactobacillus gasseri* ATCC 9857; *LJ 6, *Lactobacillus jensenii* ATCC 25258; LA cap, oral Vagiforte® capsule; LA tab, vaginal Vagiforte® tablet

4.4.3 *Lactobacillus* adhesion to Ca Ski cells

Lactobacillus adhesion to Ca Ski (ectocervical epithelial) cells was evaluated (**Figure 4.2 A-J**). It was found that the *L. acidophilus* probiotic isolate was the most adherent but interestingly, there was a large difference between the level of adhesion of the isolate obtained from the capsule (0.006%) and that of the isolate obtained from the tablet (2.022%) (**Figure 4.2A, B**). There were no statistically significant differences in adhesion between the species (**Figure 4.2A**), but among the vaginal isolates, *L. jensenii* 1 (LJ1) was the most adherent, with approximately 1.663% of bacteria adhering to the cells (**Figure 4.2B**). Several species included a relatively large proportion of highly adherent strains, with 4/6 (67%) *L. jensenii*, and 1/2 (50%), *L. gasseri* and 1/2 (50%) *L. acidophilus* relatively highly adherent. Previously, it was suggested that growth rates and bacterial size may influence the ability of the bacteria to adhere to epithelial cells (Mastromarino *et al.*, 2002). However, as observed for the isolates characterised in Chapter 3, neither the growth rates nor sizes of these isolates correlated with *Lactobacillus* adhesion (Spearman rho=0.2209, p=0.2407 and rho=0.2843, p=0.1278, respectively).

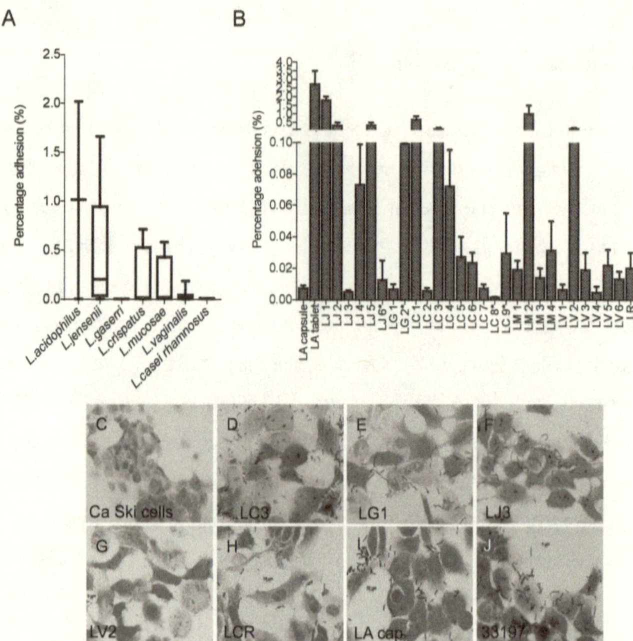

Figure 4.2: *Lactobacillus* adhesion to Ca Ski cells. (A) Adhesion was expressed as the percentage of the number of bacteria added to the monolayers that remained adherent. Species are ordered from the most to least adherent (**B**) Different isolates of the same species were grouped together. Lines indicate medians, bars indicate the interquartile ranges and error bars indicate the ranges. (**C-J**) Representative images showing lactobacilli adhesion to Ca Ski cells were taken at 1000X magnification. *Lactobacillus* isolates were cultured and adjusted to OD_{600} 0.1±0.01 in antibiotic free DMEM before being added to Ca Ski cell monolayers in chamber slides and incubated for 2 hours at 37°C with 5% CO_2. Slides were then washed to remove unbound lactobacilli and Gram stained. Representative images of the Gram stained slides were collected. LC, *Lactobacillus crispatus*; LG, *Lactobacillus gasseri*; LJ, *Lactobacillus jensenii*; LM, *Lactobacillus mucosae*; LV, *Lactobacillus vaginalis*. LC 8*, *Lactobacillus crispatus* ATCC 33197; LC 9*, *Lactobacillus crispatus* ATCC 33820; LG 2*, *Lactobacillus gasseri* ATCC 9857; LJ 6*, *Lactobacillus jensenii* ATCC 25258; LA cap, oral Vagiforte® capsule; LA tab, vaginal Vagiforte® tablet.

4.4.4 D- and L-lactate production and culture acidification

The probiotic isolates were the most acidifying in MRS broth, followed by *L. crispatus* isolates (**Figure 4.3A, B**). There was a narrow range of pH values from 3.74 up to 5.41 measured during the exponential phase of growth. *L. mucosae* and *L. vaginalis* culture pH levels were the highest. Most *Lactobacillus* isolates produced large amounts of D-lactate, but there were no significant differences between species after adjusting for multiple comparisons. (**Figure 4.3C, D**). *L. jensenii* isolates producing significantly greater amounts of L-lactate than the other isolates collectively (p=0.0013, adjusted p=0.0091), followed by *L. gasseri* and *L. vaginalis*. Interestingly, of the probiotics, only the capsule *L. acidophilus* isolate was able to produce detectable amounts of L-lactate but all three probiotic isolates produced significant amounts of D-lactate (**Figure 4.3D, F**). Total lactic acid, calculated using the Henderson-Hasselbalch equation (O'Hanlon *et al.*, 2013), correlated with culture pH (Spearman rho=0.8626, p<0.0001). A trend towards a significant correlation between D-lactate and L-lactate production was also observed (Spearman rho=0.3272, p=0.0776). Although there was a trend towards an inverse correlation between culture pH and bacterial growth rates (rho=−0.3079, p=0.0978), neither D-lactate (rho=0.07787, p=0.6825) nor L-lactate (rho=0.2520, p=0.1791) correlated with growth rates or culture pH.

D-lactate production was very similar when the lactobacilli were cultured in isolation (**Figure 4.3C, D**) compared to production by the lactobacilli in co-cultures with Ca Ski cells (**Figure 4.4A, B**). All the isolates were able to produce L-lactate in co-cultures (**Figure 4.4D**) although some of the isolates failed to produce detectable amounts in isolation (**Figure 4.3F**). Interestingly, *L. jensenii* species produced the largest concentration of D- and L-lactate in co-culture (**Figure 4.4**), and L-lactate in isolation. The probiotic isolate (*L. casei rhamnosus*) produced the least amount of L-lactate in co-culture and the least amount of both D- and L-lactate in isolation. In general, the two probiotic isolates produced lower amounts of both D and L-lactate in co-culture and in isolation compared to the vaginal isolates.

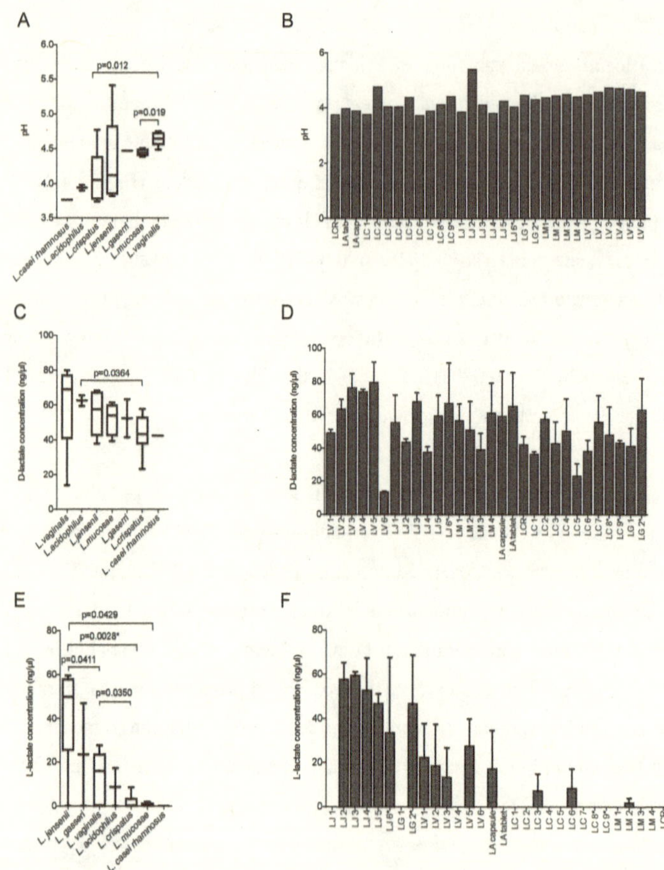

Figure 4.3: Culture acidification (pH) and D-lactate and L-lactate production by *Lactobacillus* isolates in de Man Rogosa and Sharpe (MRS) broth. (A, C, E) Tukey box plots show different strains of the same species grouped together, with the species ordered according to the magnitude of culture acidification (pH), D- and L-lactate produced. Lines indicate medians, bars indicate the interquartile ranges and error bars indicate the ranges. **(B, D, F)** Culture acidification (pH), D-lactate and L-lactate production by individual isolates are shown with bars indicating the medians and error bars indicating the ranges of technical replicates within each assay. **(C-F)** *Lactobacillus* isolates were cultured and adjusted to $4.18x10^6$ colony forming units (CFU)/ml in MRS broth then incubated for 24 hours at 37°C. Supernatants were collected and the concentrations of D-lactate, L-lactate were determined by ELISA assays. (**A, B**) Culture pH was measured using a pH meter. Mann-Whitney U test was used for comparisons between species and p-values <0.05 after adjustment for multiple comparisons were considered statistically significant. *P-values that remained statistically significant after adjustment for multiple comparisons. LC, *Lactobacillus crispatus*; LG, *Lactobacillus gasseri*; LJ, *Lactobacillus jensenii*; LM, *Lactobacillus mucosae*; LV, *Lactobacillus vaginalis*. *LC 8, *Lactobacillus crispatus* ATCC 33197; LC 9*, *Lactobacillus crispatus* ATCC 33820; LG 2*, *Lactobacillus gasseri* ATCC 9857; LJ 6*, *Lactobacillus jensenii* ATCC 25258; LA cap, oral Vagiforte® capsule; LA tab, vaginal Vagiforte® tablet.

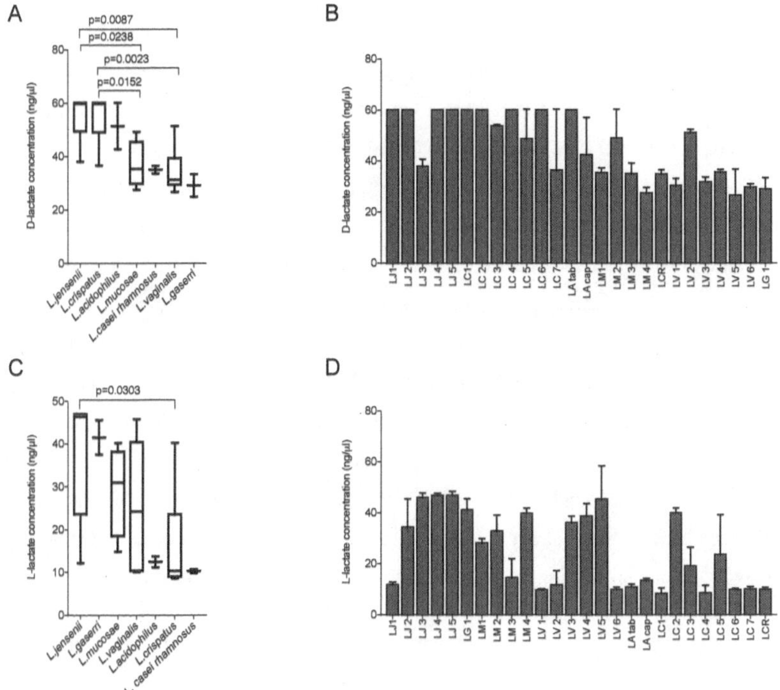

Figure 4.4: D-lactate and L-lactate production by *Lactobacillus* isolates in cell co-cultures. (A, C) Tukey box plots show different strains of the same species grouped together, with the species ordered according to D- and L-lactate production. Lines indicate medians, bars indicate the interquartile ranges and error bars indicate the ranges. (**B, D**) D-lactate and L-lactate production by individual isolates are shown with bars indicating the medians and error bars indicating the ranges of technical replicates within each assay. *Lactobacillus* isolates were cultured and adjusted to 4.18×10^6 colony forming units (CFU)/ml in antibiotic free cell culture medium and added to Ca Ski cell monolayers then incubated for 24 hours at 37°C. Supernatants were collected and the concentrations of D-lactate and L-lactate were determined by ELISA assays. LC, *Lactobacillus crispatus*; LG, *Lactobacillus gasseri*; LJ, *Lactobacillus jensenii*; LM, *Lactobacillus mucosae*; LV, *Lactobacillus vaginalis*. *LC 8, *Lactobacillus crispatus* ATCC 33197; *LC 9, *Lactobacillus crispatus* ATCC 33820; *LG 2, *Lactobacillus gasseri* ATCC 9857; *LJ 6, *Lactobacillus jensenii* ATCC 25258; LA cap, oral Vagiforte® capsule; LA tab, vaginal Vagiforte® tablet.

4.4.5 Probiotic-relevant performance of *Lactobacillus* isolates

A scoring system was formulated in order to compare and rank the lactobacilli based on the characteristics analysed. Each isolate was given a score with a maximum of three per characteristic analysed, including (1) level of adhesion to epithelial cells; the levels of (2) D-, (3) L-lactate produced, (4) growth rates and (5) culture acidification (pH) and size as described in Chapter 2 (**Table 4.2**). The *L. jensenii* strain (LJ5) ranked highest with a score of 16/18, performing better than the probiotic isolates (*L. acidophilus* and *L. casei rhamnosus*). Interestingly, the top 10 isolates included 3 *L. jensenii*, 3 *L. crispatus*, *1 L. gasseri* strain the 2 *L. acidophilus* probiotic isolates and 1 *L. vaginalis* isolate. The commercial vaginal probiotics were ranked joint 2nd with an *L. jensenii* isolate (LA tablet; 14/18), joint 4th with two *L. crispatus* isolates (LA capsule; 12/18) and joint 5th with three other isolates (LCR; 11/18). The *L. acidophilus* (capsule and tablet) strains both grew rapidly and lowered the culture pH levels effectively, but the *L. acidophilus* capsule isolate was poorly adherent to Ca Ski cells, while the *L. acidophilus* (tablet) produced very little L-lactate. Of the probiotics, the LCR probiotic strain performed the worst with poor adhesion to epithelial cells and low D- and L-lactate production in comparison to clinical isolates (**Table 4.2**).

Table 4.2: Probiotic-relevant characteristics of vaginal lactobacilli, ATCC reference strains and commercial probiotics

Sample names	Adhesion	Growth rates	Culture pH	D-lactate	L-lactate	Size	Total score
LJ 5	3	3	2	2	3	3	16
LJ 1	3	3	3	2	0	3	14
LA tab	3	3	2	3	0	3	14
LC 6	2	3	3	0	2	3	13
LA cap	1	2	3	2	2	2	12
LC 7	1	3	3	2	0	3	12
LC 1	3	3	3	0	0	3	12
LJ 4	2	3	3	0	3	0	11
LG 2*	3	0	2	2	3	1	11
LV 2	3	2	0	3	2	1	11
LCR	2	3	3	1	0	2	11
LM 2	3	2	1	1	2	1	10
LV 3	2	3	0	3	2	0	10
LV 5	2	1	0	3	3	1	10
LC 3	3	0	2	1	2	2	10
LJ 6*	1	0	2	3	3	0	9
LJ 3	1	0	2	3	3	0	9
LC 8*	1	2	2	1	0	3	9
LC 4	3	1	2	1	0	2	9
LJ 2	3	1	0	1	3	0	8
LM1	2	1	1	2	0	2	8
LV 1	1	1	1	1	2	2	8
LM 4	2	2	1	2	0	0	7
LC 9*	1	2	1	1	0	2	7
LC 2	1	2	0	2	0	2	7
LV 4	1	1	0	3	0	2	7
LM 3	2	1	1	0	0	1	5
LC 5	2	0	1	0	0	1	4
LG 1	1	0	1	0	0	2	4
LV 6	2	0	0	0	0	1	3

*ATCC reference strains; LC, *Lactobacillus crispatus*; LJ, *Lactobacillus jensenii*; LM, *Lactobacillus mucosae*; LG, *Lactobacillus gasseri*; LV, *Lactobacillus vaginalis*; LA tab, *Lactobacillus acidophilus* probiotic; LA cap, *Lactobacillus acidophilus* capsule probiotic;

4.5 Discussion

BV is highly prevalent and there are currently no effective treatment strategies (Bradshaw *et al.*, 2006; Masson *et al.*, 2014). The standard-of-care has been associated with high recurrence rates partly due to emergence of antimicrobial resistance to antibiotics (Gupta *et al.*, 1999; Cai *et al.*, 2012). Probiotics used as complementary treatment, may improve treatment outcomes by re-populating the FGT with lactobacilli species associated with health. However, the results of clinical trials investigating probiotic administration for BV treatment have been heterogenous, with some studies showing improved treatment outcomes and others showing no benefit (Bisanz *et al.*, 2014; Bohbot *et al.*, 2018; Bradshaw *et al.*, 2012; Hemalatha *et al.*, 2012; Ling *et al.*, 2013; Machado *et al.*, 2016; Paola Mastromarino *et al.*, 2009; Rapisarda *et al.*, 2018; Verdenelli *et al.*, 2016). These outcomes may be influenced by differences in the protective characteristics between probiotic strains and species (Osset *et al.*, 2001; Sanders, 2008). In this Chapter, a scoring system was developed in order to compare probiotic relevant characteristics between vaginal lactobacilli obtained from the FGTs of young South African women, ATCC reference strains and commercial probiotics. Interestingly, the vaginal lactobacilli generally performed better than the probiotics according to the criteria used here, which included lactate production, growth rates, culture acidification and adhesion to Ca Ski cells.

The species analysed in this Chapter included *L. crispatus*, *L. jensenii*, *L. mucosae*, *L. vaginalis* and *L. gasseri*, isolated from South African women. In Chapter 3, additional species including *L. johnsonii, L. plantarum, L. ruminis* and *L. salivarius* were also isolated from the genital samples. *L. iners* was not included in this analysis as it has been associated with increased risk of developing BV in women (Verstraelen *et al.*, 2009). The lactobacilli species isolated from the probiotics included *L. casei rhamnosus* and *L. acidophilus* but interestingly, none of these species were isolated from the South African women included here. This suggests that there might be a need to improve existing probiotic formulations to include species normally isolated from the FGT.

L-lactate is produced by both bacteria and vaginal cells and D-lactate is produced mostly by bacteria (Witkin *et al.*, 2013). There was a difference in L-lactate production between strains cultured in isolation and those in co-culture. It is likely that the lower L-lactate concentrations observed in the Ca Ski co-cultures is due to reduced lactobacilli growth in the cell culture media.

A limitation of the co-culture experiment was that the co-cultures were also incubated aerobically which may have influenced the lactobacilli growth, metabolism and viability (Angelis *et al.*, 2016). However, L-lactate production by the Ca Ski cells on their own was evaluated and this value was subtracted when calculating the final concentrations. It has also been shown that lactic acid produced in the FGT at physiological concentrations creates an acidic environment that inhibits BV-associated bacteria without affecting lactobacilli (O'Hanlon *et al.*, 2011). L-lactate has virucidal activity against HIV, while D-lactate was found to be inhibitory against *C. trachomatis* (Gong *et al.*, 2014). All the isolates analysed here produced detectable amounts of D-lactate. However, production of L-lactate was highly varied among the different species included in this Chapter, showing that the concentration of lactic acid in the FGT may be highly dependent on the predominant species present. Contrary to the findings of a previous study that showed that L-Lactic acid production by *L. jensenii* isolates to be below the detection level (Witkin *et al.*, 2013), *L. jensenii* isolates produced the largest amounts of L-lactate in this Chapter as well as D-lactate in Chapter 3. The vaginal lactobacilli produced more lactic acid both in co-culture with Ca Ski cells and in isolation compared to the probiotic *Lactobacillus* isolates, suggesting that the probiotics may be less protective than the vaginal lactobacilli (Witkin *et al.*, 2013). Interestingly, both the *L. acidophilus* tablet and *L. casei rhamnosus* did not produce detectable amounts of L-lactate, further supporting the importance of thoroughly evaluating candidate probiotics to improve the formulations.

The isolates analysed in this Chapter were able to acidify culture medium to a range that closely matches that seen in *Lactobacillus*-dominated FGTs (Boskey *et al.*, 1999). During BV, the vaginal pH rises as vaginal lactobacilli are lost and overgrowth of diverse bacteria occurs. Similar to previous findings (O'Hanlon *et al.*, 2013), the current study found that culture pH correlated negatively with lactic acid production by the lactobacilli, supporting the notion that lactobacilli play a critical role in acidification in the FGT. Interestingly, despite producing relatively little lactic acid, the *L. casei rhamnosus* and *L. acidophilus* probiotics acidified the culture medium the most compared to the vaginal isolates.

The adhesion of lactobacilli to the genital epithelium has been described as the first step in the formation of a barrier to prevent undesirable microbial colonization, enabling the lactobacilli to persist in the FGT (Boris *et al*., 1998; Atassi *et al*., 2006). In the current study, the *L. acidophilus* probiotic was the most adherent, although the differences observed between species analysed here were not statistically significant. In Chapter 3, *L. jensenii* isolates were the most adherent when compared to the other lactobacilli species. Persistence of lactobacilli in the FGT was not evaluated but previous studies have found that *Lactobacillus* strains included in probiotic formulations were only detectable for the duration of the treatment, with the majority showing a decrease within weeks after treatment cessation, suggesting failure to persist in the FGT (Gardiner *et al*., 2002; Burton *et al*, 2003; Antonio *et al*., 2009; Ehrström *et al*., 2010; Bisanz *et al*., 2014; Tomusiak *et al*., 2015; Verdenelli *et al*., 2016; van de Wijgert *et al*., 2019). Further studies need to be carried out to assess and improve lactobacilli persistence in the FGT. Evidence of viability of the lactobacilli may also be an indication of persistence in the FGT and may be correlated to production of protective metabolites (Gueimonde *et al*., 2006). In the current study, viability was not evaluated but all of the lactobacilli isolates analysed, including the probiotics, showed active growth, with marked variation between strains. However, the production of D- nor L-lactate metabolites did not correlate with lactobacilli growth rates. Interestingly, there is evidence of poor viability or dormant bacteria in commercial formulations, suggesting the need for more improved formulations and storage conditions (Ravula *et al*., 1998; Amor *et al*., 2002; Lahtinen *et al*., 2005; Lahtinen *et al*., 2006). Adhesion was not associated with size or growth rates in this Chapter as previously suggested (Mastromarino *et al*., 2002). A limitation of this analysis was that a small sample size of lactobacilli isolates was used and very few vaginal probiotics were commercially available in South Africa. It is worth noting that there is need to evaluate lactobacilli antibiotic resistance as well as non-invasiveness in epithelial cell lines to ensure safety (Gueimonde & Salminen, 2006). Furthermore, dose-response assessments to determine the optimal quantity of lactobacilli for a given probiotic formulation are also important (Atassi *et al*., 2006; Hütt *et al*., 2016).

The findings in this Chapter show that some vaginal isolates performed better than isolates obtained from the commercial probiotics that were included here. The results also show variations in probiotic-relevant characteristics both between lactobacilli strains and species. Additionally the lactobacilli isolated from these commercial probiotics were not among the species isolated from the FGTs of the women described in this Chapter, as well as Chapter 3. This supports the need for novel probiotic formulations including fully characterised *Lactobacillus* species that are normally found in the FGT in order to improve BV treatment outcomes.

CHAPTER 5: *Lactobacillus*-mediated modulation of HIV pseudovirus infectivity in TZM-bl cells

5.1 Summary

The majority of the HIV infections in women are acquired via the FGT epithelium. In women with optimal microbiota, the vaginal epithelium is mostly colonised by *Lactobacillus*-dominated species. Disturbances in the vaginal microbiota that result in the depletion of *Lactobacillus* species have been associated with the upregulation of proinflammatory cytokines and increased susceptibility to HIV acquisition. While a *Lactobacillus*-dominated vaginal microbiota is associated with reduced HIV risk, the relative importance of different *Lactobacillus* species has not been defined. The aim of this Chapter was to compare the effects of different cervicovaginal *Lactobacillus* species on HIV pseudovirus infectivity. Vaginal *Lactobacillus* isolates (n=16), including *L. crispatus* (n=4), *L. jensenii* (n=4), *L. mucosae* (n=4) and *L. vaginalis* (n=4), were isolated from young South African women with optimal microbiota (n=8) and women with non-optimal microbiota (n=8), who participated in the Women's Initiative in Sexual Health (WISH) study. The influence of the *Lactobacillus* culture supernatants on HIV infectivity was evaluated using a Luciferase Reporter Gene Assay in TZM-bl cells. The ability of vaginal *Lactobacillus* to produce lactic acid and acidify cultures, and their sizes, adhesion to epithelial cells and growth rates were also evaluated to determine possible underlying mechanisms for changes in HIV infectivity. All 16 lactobacilli isolates analysed here suppressed pseudovirus entry with *L. crispatus* and *L. vaginalis* isolates inhibiting entry to the greatest degree (p=0.0044) followed by *L. jensenii* isolates (p=0.0308), although a large variation was observed between the strains. No significant differences were observed in *Lactobacillus* sizes, growth rates, adhesion to vaginal epithelial cells or production of D/L-lactate while culture acidification correlated with HIV pseudovirus infectivity (Spearman rho=0.5471; p=0.0283). Overall, these findings suggest that *Lactobacillus* species may suppress HIV infectivity in a strain-specific manner. Additionally, these findings may be an important step towards development of strategies that women can control themselves such as topical biotherapeutics to help reduce HIV acquisition in order to improve their genital health.

5.2 Introduction

HIV transmission from infected to uninfected individuals can occur across mucosal surfaces through unprotected sexual intercourse, exchange of body fluids, sharing of needles during injection drug use or vertically through mother-to-child transmission (Pope & Haase, 2003; Correa and Gisselquist, 2006; Anderson *et al.*, 2011; Shaw & Hunter, 2012). Heterosexual transmission is the predominant mode of transmission worldwide accounting for the majority of all HIV-1 infections (Simon *et al.*, 2006; UNAIDS, 2016). Transmission rates are said to be greater from males to females than vice versa (UNAIDS, 2014; Gosmann *et al.*, 2017), highlighting the importance of understanding the FGT and HIV acquisition. Interestingly, the risk of HIV acquisition via the FGT mucosa is said to be lower than rectal or parenteral transmission (Powers *et al.*, 2008), potentially due to antimicrobial and innate immune system defense mechanisms in the FGT, as well as protective compounds produced by commensal bacteria (Soledad *et al.*, 2000; Cone, 2008; Lai *et al.*, 2009). However, transmission risk strongly correlates with HIV viral load in the infected individuals (Marks *et al.*, 2016). Women in resource limited settings have limited means to actively protect themselves against HIV infection, especially since there are no known effective vaccines (Chang *et al.*, 2003). Development of an effective vaccine has proved challenging due to the degree of genetic diversity of HIV-1 and structural complexity of its envelope glycoprotein (Env) (Wyatt and Sodroski, 1998; Kwong *et al.*, 2002). Other studies have investigated the use of topical microbicides, however efficacy is limited and certain antiretroviral microbicides lack effectiveness in women with upregulated inflammatory cytokine levels in the FGT or non-optimal microbiota (Abdool Karim *et al.*, 2010; Klatt *et al.*, 2017; McKinnon *et al.*, 2018). Topical pre-exposure prophylaxis has been found to be highly efficacious, however some studies have reported poor adherence (Van Der Straten *et al.*, 2012; Marrazzo *et al.*, 2015; Atujuna *et al.*, 2018). Therefore, there is urgent need for the development of alternative methods of HIV prevention, the use of which is controlled by women.

Evidently, the cervicovaginal epithelium is a key site for HIV entry in women for a productive infection (Kaushic *et al.*, 2010). In women with optimal microbiota, the vaginal epithelium is mostly colonised by *Lactobacillus*-dominated species (Antonio *et al.*, 1999; Anukam *et al.*, 2005; Burton *et al.*, 2003; Ravel *et al.*, 2011). Disturbances in the vaginal microbiota that result in the depletion of *Lactobacillus* species have been associated with the development of BV and increased susceptibility to infections, leading to an upregulation of proinflammatory cytokines (Mlisana *et al*., 2012; Masson *et al*., 2014; Eastment *et al*., 2015; Lennard *et al*., 2017). Inflammation is critical for maintaining health in the FGT and clearing infections, however the presence of inflammatory cytokines in the FGT prior to HIV exposure also increases susceptibility to HIV acquisition (Masson *et al*., 2015). HIV acquisition risk increases likely by recruitment of activated HIV target cells, such as CD4+ T-cells, to the vaginal mucosal epithelium, promotion of HIV transcription via nuclear factor kappa B (NF-κB) activation and disruption of the integrity of the epithelial barrier (Osborn *et al*., 1989; Doerflinger., 2014; Masson *et al*., 2015; Anahtar *et al*., 2015; Arnold *et al*., 2016; Klatt *et al*., 2017).

As lactobacilli are associated with reduced levels of inflammatory cytokines production in the FGT (Lennard *et al*., 2017), and fewer numbers of activated CD4+ T cells compared to those with BV-associated bacteria (BVAB)-dominated microbiomes (Gosmann *et al*., 2017), colonisation with *Lactobacillus* spp. may reduce susceptibility to HIV acquisition in women. Studies have shown that the majority of South African women have *Lactobacillus*-deficient vaginal microbiomes and are thus at an increased risk of STI infection, including HIV (Gosmann *et al*., 2017; Lennard *et al*., 2017; Ravel *et al*., 2011). Although it has been shown that cervicovaginal bacteria modulate genital inflammation, their role in HIV susceptibility is not yet fully understood. Gosmann *et al* also showed that women with *L. crispatus*-dominated FGTs were at the lowest risk of HIV acquisition compared to those with diverse genital bacterial communities (Gosmann *et al*., 2017).

To investigate the effect of cervicovaginal *Lactobacillus* isolates on HIV infectivity, TZM-bl cells were exposed to HIV pseudovirus in the presence or absence of lactobacilli conditioned culture medium. The ability of vaginal *Lactobacillus* to produce lactic acid and acidify cultures, and their sizes, adhesion to epithelial cells and growth rates were also evaluated to determine possible underlying mechanisms for changes in HIV infectivity.

5.3 Methods

5.3.1 Study cohort and sample selection

This Chapter included 16 *Lactobacillus* isolates (8 from BV negative women and 8 from BV positive women). The 16 isolates analysed in this Chapter were different from those analysed in Chapter 4 to further investigate a trend observed in the 23 vaginal isolates in Chapter 4 suggesting that isolates obtained from women with BV were associated with greater inflammatory responses when co-cultured with epithelial cells. Growth rates, bacterial sizes, adhesion to VK2 cells, culture pH changes and D/L-lactate production by the lactobacilli were also measured *in vitro*. HIV pseudovirus was prepared by co-transfecting HEK293T cells with Env expression plasmid and an Env-deficient HIV-1 backbone vector (pSG3Δenv), using polyethylenimine (PEI) transfection agent. The pseudovirus aliquots with the highest infectivity were selected for technical replicates and the experiment was conducted 3 times. The influence of the *Lactobacillus* culture supernatants on the HIV pseudovirus infectivity in TZM-bl cells containing Tat-responsive reporter genes for firefly luciferase and expressing CD4, CXCR4, and CCR5 was evaluated using a Luciferase Reporter Gene Assay as described in Chapter 2.

5.4 Results

5.4.1 Study population and description of vaginal *Lactobacillus* isolates

A total of 16 *Lactobacillus* isolates comprising *L. crispatus* (n=4), *L. jensenii* (n=4), *L. mucosae* (n=4) and *L. vaginalis* (n=4) were analysed in this Chapter. Eight of the isolates were obtained from BV negative (Nugent score 0-3) women and the other eight from BV positive women (Nugent score 7-10). The median age of the women was 18 years (range 16-22) and all of the women were taking progesterone-based contraceptives at the time of sample collection. Four of the women had *C. trachomatis* infections, one had a *N. gonorrhoeae* infection, one had a *T. vaginalis* infection, one was shedding HSV-2 and one participant was coinfected with *N. gonorrhoeae, T. vaginalis and C. trachomatis* infections. At the time of sampling, none of the participants tested positive for *T. pallidum* or had yeast infections.

5.4.2 Description of baseline characteristics of vaginal *Lactobacillus* isolates

5.4.2.1 Baseline number of colony forming units in cultures standardised to OD_{600} 0.1$\pm$0.01

The baseline characteristics of the *Lactobacillus* isolates were evaluated. All isolates were normalised to OD_{600} 0.1$\pm$0.01 and CFUs were counted to allow for standardisation of each culture prior to each experiment. All of the isolates analysed were viable on MRS agar plates shown by the presence of multiple colonies (**Figure 5.1A**) and showed the characteristic creamy or milky white, round and opaque colonies. There was however variation in the number of CFUs between the species, although the differences were not statistically significant. *L. mucosae* isolates had the highest CFUs while *L. jensenii* isolates had the least CFUs (**Figure 5.1B**).

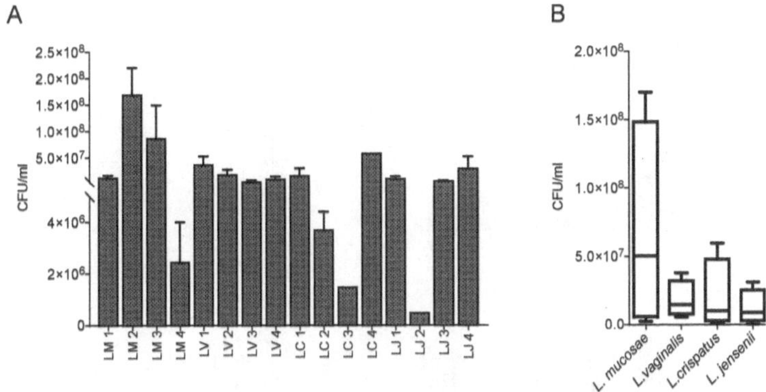

Figure 5.1: Number of colony forming units (CFU)/ml in standardized cultures of lactobacilli isolates. (**A**) Lactobacilli CFU/ml for individual isolates. Data are shown as medians with ranges. (**B**) Lactobacilli (CFU/ml) grouped by species. Lactobacilli including [*L. crispatus* (n=4), *L. jensenii* (n=4), *L. mucosae* (n=4) and *L. vaginalis* (n=4)] were cultured in de Man Rogosa and Sharpe (MRS) broth, adjusted to an optical density (OD) at 600nm of 0.1±0.01, serially diluted and then plated on MRS agar plates in triplicate. Following incubation for 24 hours under anaerobic conditions, CFUs were manually counted and CFU/ml calculated for each isolate. Mann Whitney U tests were used to compare CFUs between different lactobacilli species and p-values were adjusted for multiple comparisons using a false discovery rate step-down procedure. No statistically significant differences ($p<0.05$) were observed. LC, *Lactobacillus crispatus*; LJ, *Lactobacillus jensenii*; LM, *Lactobacillus mucosae*; LV, *Lactobacillus vaginalis*.

5.4.2.2 *Lactobacillus* growth rates, bacterial sizes and adhesion to vaginal epithelial cells

Although no significant differences were observed in *Lactobacillus* sizes between species, *L. vaginalis* isolates were the smallest and *L. crispatus* were the largest compared to the other species (**Figure 5.2A,B**). Growth rates were highly varied between strains as expected (**Figure 5.2C**). *L. crispatus* isolates grew most rapidly, followed by *L. vaginalis* isolates, *L. mucosae* and then *L. jensenii* isolates (**Figure 5.2D**), although the differences observed were not statistically significant. *L. jensenii* isolates were the most adherent while *L. vaginalis* isolates were the least adherent to vaginal epithelial cells (**Figure 5.2E,F**). However, there was no correlation between size and CFUs/ml in standardized cultures (Spearman rho=-0.3938, p=0.1313; **Figure 5.3**).

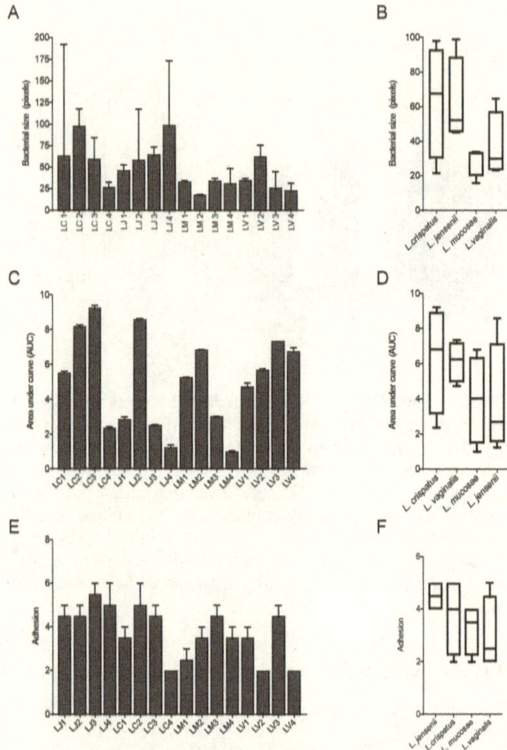

Figure 5.2: Bacterial sizes, growth rates and adhesion. (A,C,E,) Characteristics of individual isolates. **(B,D,F)** Characteristics shown by species. (**A,B**) Single colonies were picked from *Lactobacillus* cultures [*L. crispatus* (n=4), *L. jensenii* (n=4), *L. mucosae* (n=4) and *L. vaginalis* (n=4)], and smears were prepared on microscope slides and Gram-stained before collecting images at 1000X magnification. Bacterial size was determined from the images using Image J^{TM} software. Bacterial sizes were calculated as the mean of five measurements. (**C,D**) Lactobacilli isolates were cultured and adjusted to 4.18×10^6 colony forming units (CFU)/ml, inoculated into 96-well plates in triplicate, before incubating anaerobically and measuring the optical density (OD_{600nm}) at six time points 3 hours apart from baseline up to 24 hours. Growth rates were determined in triplicate and the graphs show the area under curve (AUC) for each isolate and by species as determined in GraphPad Prism. (**E,F**) *Lactobacillus* isolates were cultured and adjusted to 4.18×10^6 CFU/ml in antibiotic free keratinocyte serum free media before being added to VK2 cell monolayers in chamber slides and incubated for 2 hours at 37°C with 5% CO_2. Slides were then washed to remove unbound lactobacilli and Gram-stained. Representative images of the Gram-stained slides were collected and *Lactobacillus* isolates were ranked according to level of adhesion in ascending order from least adherent (**1**) to most adherent (**6**). The level of adhesion was determined in duplicate. **(A,C,E,)** Bars indicate medians and error bars indicate ranges. **(B,D,F)** Tukey box plots show different strains of the same species grouped together, with the species ordered according to sizes, growth rates and adhesion. Lines indicate medians, bars indicate the interquartile ranges and error bars indicate the ranges. Mann-Whitney U test was used for comparisons between species and p-values <0.05 after adjustment for multiple comparisons were considered statistically significant. LC, *Lactobacillus crispatus*; LJ, *Lactobacillus jensenii*; LM, *Lactobacillus mucosae*; LV, *Lactobacillus vaginalis*.

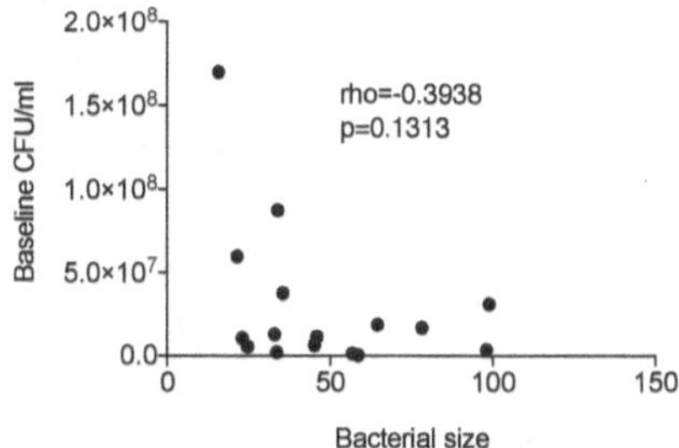

Figure 5.3: Correlation between baseline colony forming units (CFU)/ml and bacterial size. Lactobacilli [*L. crispatus* (n=4), *L. jensenii* (n=4), *L. mucosae* (n=4) and *L. vaginalis* (n=4)] were cultured in de Man Rogosa and Sharpe (MRS) broth, adjusted to an optical density (OD) at 600nm 0.1$\pm$0.01, serially diluted and then plated on MRS agar plates in triplicate. Following incubation for 24 hours under anaerobic conditions, CFUs were manually counted and CFU/ml calculated for each isolate. Single colonies were picked from *Lactobacillus* cultures smears were prepared on microscope slides and Gram-stained before collecting images at 1000X magnification. Bacterial size was determined from the images using Image J^{TM} software. There was no correlation between size and baseline CFUs (Spearman rho=-0.3938, p=0.1313).

5.4.2.3 D and L-lactate production by vaginal *Lactobacillus* isolates and culture acidification

All of the lactobacilli isolates were able to produce detectable amounts of D and L-lactate in culture supernatants (**Figure 5.4A-D**). While there were no statistically significant differences in D- and L-lactate production and cultures pH between species, collectively, *L. crispatus* isolates produced the highest concentration of D-lactate while *L. mucosae* isolates produced the lowest concentration in culture. However, *L. mucosae* isolates produced the most L-lactate followed by *L. jensenii*, *L. vaginalis* and *L. crispatus*. *L. crispatus* isolates produced the greatest concentration of total lactic acid in culture (**Figure 5.4E,F**). Culture pH values ranged between 3.84 and 4.56 (**Figure 5.4G,H**), corresponding with the expected vaginal pH in women with an optimal vaginal microbiota. *L. vaginalis* isolates acidified culture medium the most, followed by *L. mucosae*, *L. jensenii* and *L. crispatus*. Neither L-lactate (Spearman rho=-0.2412), p=0.3669, D-lactate (Spearman rho=-0.1353, p=0.6170), while total lactic acid (Spearman rho=-0.8412, p<0.0001) strongly correlated with culture acidification (**Figure 5.5A-C**).

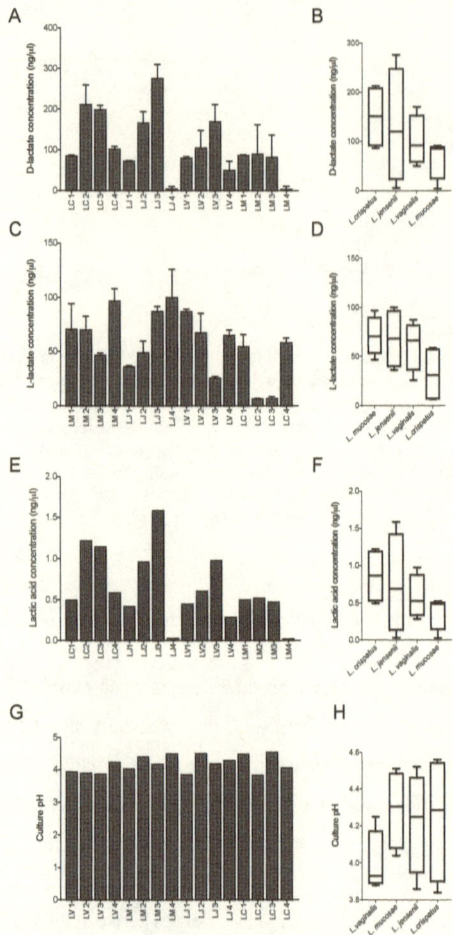

Figure 5.4: D-lactate and L-lactate production, total lactic acid and culture acidification (pH) by *Lactobacillus* isolates. **(A,C)** D-lactate and L-lactate production by individual isolates are shown with bars indicating the medians and error bars indicating the ranges of technical replicates within each assay. **(E,G)** Single pH measurements were collected and thus total lactic acid was calculated using the median of D- and L-lactate concentrations. **(B,D,F,H)** Characteristics of lactobacilli grouped according to species. Lactobacilli isolates [*L. crispatus* (n=4), *L. jensenii* (n=4), *L. mucosae* (n=4) and *L. vaginalis* (n=4)] were cultured and adjusted to 4.18×10^6 colony forming units (CFU)/ml in de Man Rogosa and Sharpe (MRS) broth then incubated anaerobically for 24 hours at 37°C. Supernatants were collected and the concentrations of D-lactate and L-lactate were determined by ELISA assays. Culture pH was measured using a pH meter. Lines indicate medians, bars indicate the interquartile ranges and error bars indicate the ranges. Mann-Whitney U test was used for comparisons between species and p-values <0.05 after adjustment for multiple comparisons were considered statistically significant. LC, *Lactobacillus crispatus*; LJ, *Lactobacillus jensenii*; LM, *Lactobacillus mucosae*; LV, *Lactobacillus vaginalis*.

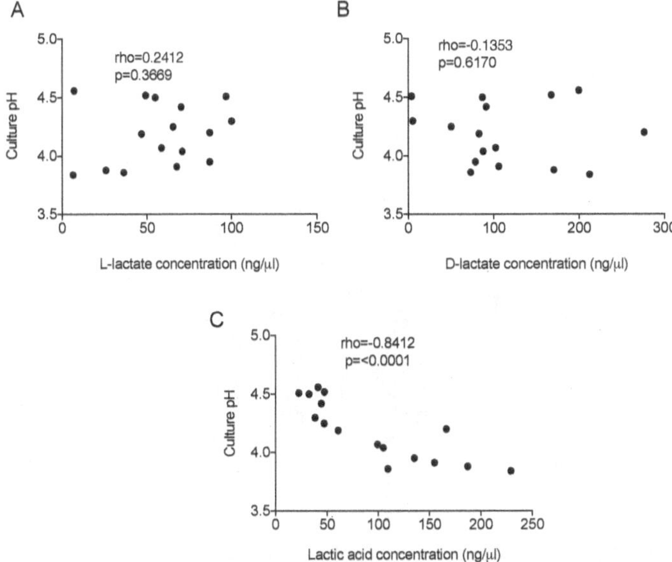

Figure 5.5: Correlation between culture pH and L-lactate, D-lactate and lactic acid concentration. (**A**) Correlation between culture pH and L-lactate concentration (Spearman rho=0.2412, p=03669) (**B**) Correlation between culture pH and D-lactate concentration (Spearman rho=-0.1353, p=0.6170). (**C**) Correlation between culture pH and lactic acid concentration (Spearman rho=-0.1353, p=0.6170). *Lactobacillus* isolates (n=16) were cultured and adjusted to 4.18x10^{6} colony forming units (CFU)/ml in MRS broth then incubated for 24 hours at 37°C. Supernatants were collected and the concentrations of D-lactate, L-lactate were determined in duplicate by ELISA assays. Total lactic acid was calculated using the Henderson-Hasselbach formula. Culture pH was measured using a pH meter.

5.4.3 HIV pseudovirus infectivity in TZM-bl cells

To determine the HIV-1 inhibitory activity of vaginal *Lactobacillus* isolates, conditioned culture medium collected from vaginal lactobacilli cultures was incubated with HIV pseudovirus and assayed for infectivity using TZM-bl indicator cells in an assay that allows measurement of a single round of HIV-1 infection. Pseudovirus standardized by p24 ELISA to 200ng/μl in complete DMEM was added to TZM-bl cells in the presence of lactobacilli conditioned culture medium. All the pseudovirus analysed here was able to successfully enter TZM-bl cells. All the lactobacilli isolates analysed suppressed HIV pseudovirus infectivity to levels below that of the control which contained MRS broth only with varying levels of suppression between strains. (**Figure 5.6**).

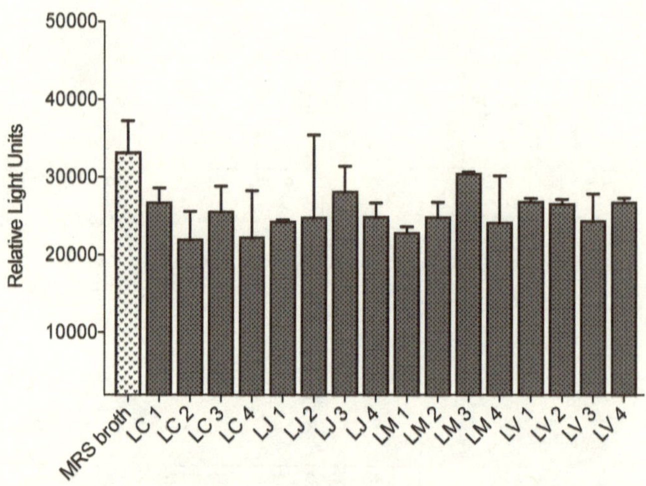

Figure 5.6: Comparison of the inhibitory activities of *Lactobacillus* strains towards HIV pseudovirus. *Lactobacillus* strains (n=16) in de Man Rogosa and Sharpe (MRS) broth for 24 hours at 37°C and adjusted to 4.18×10^6 colony forming units (CFU)/ml before collecting conditioned medium from the cultures. TZM-bl cells were seeded at 1×10^4 cells/well in a 96 well tissue culture plates and incubated at 37°C with 5% CO_2 for 24 hours. HIV pseudovirus at a concentration of 200ng/μl was added in triplicate to the TZM-bl cells and incubated at 37°C with 5% CO_2 in the presence or absence of 10μl of conditioned lactobacilli culture medium with a pseudovirus-only control well with only MRS broth added. Bars indicate median values of the relative light units with standard error bars indicating standard deviation determined in three independent experiments shown. A one-way ANOVA with Tukey post-tests showed no significant differences. LC, *Lactobacillus crispatus*; LJ, *Lactobacillus jensenii*; LM, *Lactobacillus mucosae*; LV, *Lactobacillus vaginalis*.

When the absolute level of infectivity was compared, it was found that all the lactobacilli species analysed were able to suppress pseudovirus entry with *L. crispatus* (p=0.0044), *L. vaginalis* (p=0.0044) and *L. jensenii* (p=0.0308) isolates demonstrating significant suppression, however suppression by *L. jensenii* was not statistically significant after adjusting for multiple comparisons (**Figure 5.7A**). Conditioned culture medium from lactobacilli isolates obtained from both women with optimal (p=0.0072) and those with non-optimal (p=0.0212) microbiota suppressed pseudovirus entry (**Figure 5.7B**). Overall, all of the lactobacilli isolates suppressed pseudovirus entry significantly (p=0.0078; **Figure 5.7C**).

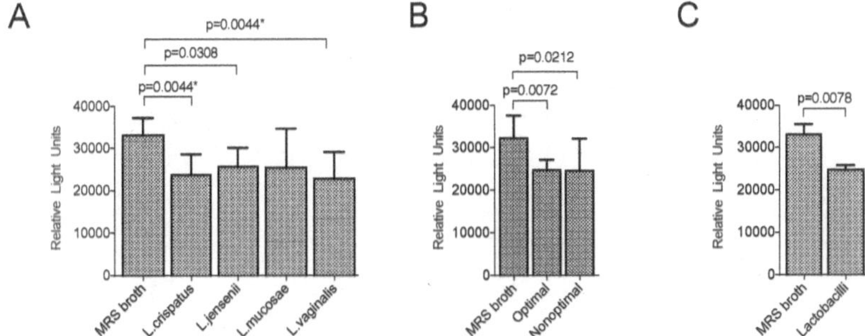

Figure 5.7: Effect of lactobacilli conditioned culture medium on HIV pseudovirus infectivity in TZM-bl cells. (A) Effect of conditioned medium shown in isolates grouped by species. (**B**) Comparison of the effect of conditioned culture medium from lactobacilli obtained from women with optimal (Nugent 0-3; n=8) and women with BV (Nugent 7-10; n=8). **(C)** Overall effect of conditioned culture medium from all lactobacilli (n=16) on pseudovirus infectivity. TZM-bl cells were seeded at $1x10^4$ cells/well in a 96 well tissue culture plate and incubated at 37°C with 5% CO_2 for 24 hours. HIV pseudovirus at a concentration of 200ng/µl was added in triplicate to the TZM-bl cells and incubated at 37°C with 5% CO_2 in the presence or absence of 10µl of conditioned lactobacilli culture medium with a pseudovirus-only control well with only MRS broth added. Bars show the median and ranges. Mann Whitney U tests were used for comparisons and p-values <0.05 after adjustment for multiple comparisons were considered statistically significant.

5.3.4 Correlation between HIV pseudovirus infectivity and lactobacilli characteristics

To investigate the factors that may be influencing pseudovirus infectivity, Spearman correlations between lactobacilli characteristics and pseudovirus infectivity were evaluated. HIV infectivity was positively correlated with culture pH, suggesting that lower pH ranges were likely to inhibit HIV infectivity (Spearman rho=0.5471; p=0.0283; **Figure 5.8A**), Lactobacilli adhesion to vaginal epithelial cells (Spearman rho=0.1886; p=4803), D-lactate production (Spearman rho=0.1; p=0.7132), L-lactate production (Spearman rho=0.15; p=0.5786) and lactic acid concentration (Spearman rho=-0.3588; p=0.1727) did not correlate with HIV infectivity (**Figure 5.8B,C,D**).

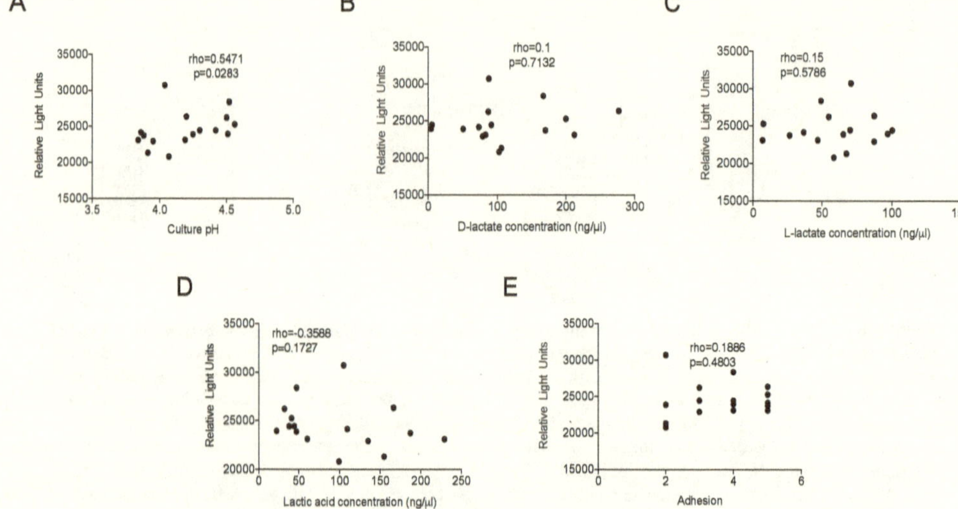

Figure 5.8: Correlation between HIV pseudovirus entry and D-lactate, L-lactate, lactic acid concentration and culture pH. (**A**) Correlation between pseudovirus entry and (**A**) culture pH (Spearman rho=0.5471; p=0.0283); (**B**) D-lactate concentration (Spearman rho=0.1; p=0.7132); (**C**) L-lactate concentration (Spearman rho=0.15; p=0.5786); (**D**) lactic acid concentration (Spearman rho=0.1; p=0.7132); (**E**) lactobacilli adhesion to VK2 cells (Spearman rho=0.1886; p=0.4803) (**A,B,C,D**) TZM-bl cells were seeded at $1x10^4$ cells/well in a 96 well tissue culture plate and incubated at 37°C with 5% CO_2 for 24 hours. HIV pseudovirus at a concentration of 200ng/μl was added in triplicate to the TZM-bl cells and incubated at 37°C with 5% CO_2 in the presence or absence of 10μl of conditioned lactobacilli culture medium with a pseudovirus-only control well with only MRS broth added. RLUs represent data from 3 biological repeats. Culture pH was measured using a pH meter. (**E**) *Lactobacillus* isolates were cultured and adjusted to $4.18x10^6$ CFU/ml in antibiotic free keratinocyte serum free media before being added to VK2 cell monolayers in chamber slides and incubated for 2 hours at 37°C with 5% CO_2. Slides were then washed to remove unbound lactobacilli and Gram-stained. Representative images of the Gram-stained slides were collected and *Lactobacillus* isolates were ranked according to level of adhesion in ascending order from least adherent (**1**) to most adherent (**6**).

5.4 Discussion

The predominant mode of HIV transmission is via heterosexual contact and the cervicovaginal epithelium is the key site for HIV entry in women (Chang *et al.*, 2003; Hladik and Hope, 2019). Young women in developing countries are at an exceptionally high risk of HIV acquisition due to social, behavioural and structural factors (Harrison *et al.*, 2015; Chang *et al.*, 2003). Since a *Lactobacillus*-dominated vaginal microbiota is considered optimal in the FGT and is associated with relatively low levels of inflammation as well as very low risk of HIV acquisition (Gosmann *et al.*, 2017), an *in vitro* system was used to investigate the effect of lactobacilli conditioned culture medium on HIV pseudovirus infectivity in TZM-bl cells and to compare inhibition of pseudovirus infectivity by 4 lactobacilli species including *L. crispatus*, *L. jensenii*, *L. mucosae* and *L. vaginalis*. Collectively, *L. crispatus* and *L.vaginalis* isolates significantly inhibited pseudovirus infectivity to the greatest degree while *L. crispatus* produced the greatest concentration of total lactic acid compared with the other lactobacilli species. *L. vaginalis* isolates acidified culture medium the most compared to the other species. There were no significant differences between isolates from women with optimal microbiota and those with BV. HIV infectivity was positively correlated with culture pH, but was not associated with *Lactobacillus* growth rates, adhesion to vaginal epithelial cells, or D- nor L-lactate production.

In the past, it has been reported that the presence of lactobacilli in the FGT is associated with a reduced susceptibility to HIV infection (Anahtar *et al.*, 2015; Gosmann *et al.*, 2017) and, in support to these findings, the current study suggests that *Lactobacillus* species associated with an optimal FGT microbiome (including *L. crispatus*, *L. jensenii*, *L. vaginalis* and *L. mucosae*) are able to inhibit HIV infectivity. As abiotic *Lactobacillus* culture medium was added, this inhibition was at least in part due to metabolites produced by the lactobacilli that resulted in culture acidification (Aldunate *et al.*, 2015; Hearps *et al.*, 2017; Tyssen *et al.*, 2018). A previous study showed that incubation of HIV-1 in lactobacilli conditioned medium significantly inhibited viral infectivity in human tissues *ex vivo* which correlated with lactic acid concentration (Palomino *et al.*, 2017). Greater inhibition of pseudovirus entry by *L. crispatus*-conditioned and *L. vaginalis*-conditioned medium suggests that different *Lactobacillus* species may confer different levels of protection against HIV. However, it is worth noting that the level of inhibition varied between individual strains, suggesting that inhibition may also be strain specific. Women with *L. crispatus*- dominated vaginal microbiota have also been shown to be at a lower risk of HIV acquisition than women colonized with *L. iners* (Borgdorff *et al*., 2014; Gosmann *et al*., 2017). The lack of a significant difference between isolates from women with optimal microbiota versus BV may be due to the fact that there were no differences in culture acidification between the isolates (not shown) since virucidal activity has been shown to be pH-dependent (Aldunate *et al*., 2013; Tyssen *et al*., 2018). However the sample size of this analysis was small, limiting the power to identify statistically significant differences between groups.

Lactobacillus isolates produce lactic acid which creates an acidic environment in the FGT, significantly reducing the risk of acquiring STIs (Allsworth *et al*., 2008; Kaul *et al*., 2007), including HIV (Atashili *et al*., 2008; Taha *et al*., 1998), in women or transmission of HIV to a partner (Cohen *et al*., 2012). In this Chapter, all of the lactobacilli produced detectable amounts of both D and L-lactate in culture, while *L. crispatus* isolates produced the largest amount of total lactic acid in culture. Lactic acid exists as L- and D- isomers most of which is produced by lactobacilli in the FGT (Tachedjian *et al*., 2017). L-lactic acid has been reported to be more effective at inactivating HIV than D-lactate (Aldunate *et al*., 2015) and has been shown to demonstrate potent HIV virucidal activity at physiological concentrations (Connor, 2006; Kempf & Jentsch, 1991; Martin *et al*., 1985; O'Connor *et al*., 1995; Aldunate *et al*., 2013; Tyssen *et al*., 2018). Additionally, it has also been reported that lactic acid has broad-spectrum virucidal activity against various HIV subtypes as well as transmitted/founder strains of HIV-1 in a pH-dependent manner (Aldunate *et al*., 2013; Tyssen *et al*., 2018). While L-lactic acid also has antimicrobial activity against BV-associated bacteria (Boris & Barbés, 2000; O'Hanlon *et al*., 2011; Stamey & Timothy, 1975), D-lactate is thought to have greater activity against bacterial pathogens such as chlamydia infection (Tachedjian *et al*., 2017).

The activity of lactic acid against HIV has been found to be in a pH-dependent manner (Aldunate *et al*., 2013; Tyssen *et al*., 2018). Similarly, in this Chapter pseudovirus infectivity was positively correlated with culture pH, supporting the notion that an acidic pH has a protective effect against HIV infectivity. As expected, lactic acid concentration was positively correlated with culture pH suggesting that the lactobacilli were able to acidify cultures through production of metabolites such as lactic acid. It is, however, not clear which metabolites produced by the lactobacilli were responsible for the inhibition of HIV as lactate production was not associated with HIV infectivity. Previous studies have shown also that lactic acid is the major organic acid metabolite produced by

Lactobacillus-dominated microbiota (Zalán *et al.*, 2010; Aldunate *et al.*, 2013), however it is possible that other metabolites such as acetic acid contributed to the pseudovirus inhibition. Alternatively, it is possible that the sample size in this analysis was too small to demonstrate a significant correlation between HIV infectivity and total lactic acid.

Studies have also reported that H_2O_2, which is also produced by *Lactobacillus* species, is an important microbicide that is toxic to microorganisms including HIV and HSV-2 (Conti, Malacrino, & Mastromarino, 2009; Klebanoff & Coombs, 1991). H_2O_2 is said to have virucidal effect on HIV by inhibiting viral adhesion and replication (Klebanoff & Coombs, 1991). However, H_2O_2 concentrations were not evaluated in the cultures analysed here as it has been shown that lactobacilli are unlikely to produce significant H_2O_2 under anaerobic conditions. Bacteriocins produced by lactobacilli also have microbicidal effects by permeabilizing the membranes of pathogenic Gram-negative bacteria (Danielsson *et al.*, 2011). Studies have been carried out to investigate the use of bacteriocins as antiviral agents and interestingly, some studies showed inhibitory activity against HSV-2, Influenza, Hepatitis C virus and Coxsackievirus (Serkedjieva *et al.*, 2000; Mastromarino *et al.*, 2011; Kassaa *et al.*, 2014; El-Adawi *et al.*, 2015; Arena *et al.*, 2018). However, the possibility of antiviral activity against HIV is unknown and studies have mostly looked at antiviral activity by bacteriocins from species other than lactobacilli with the bacteriocins showing antiviral activity against viruses such as HSV-1, HSV-2, poliovirus and influenza virus (Férir *et al.*, 2013; Qureshi *et al.*, 2006; Saeed *et al.*, 2007; Todorov *et al.*, 2010, 2005; Torres *et al.*, 2013; Wachsman *et al.*, 2003; Cavicchioli *et al.*, 2018).

Overall, these findings suggest that the presence of *Lactobacillus* species in the FGT may protect against HIV infection in a species-specific manner as previously reported (Tyssen *et al.*, 2018). However, the variation observed between different strains may also suggest that the level of protection is strain-specific. Additionally, these findings may be an important step towards development of strategies to help reduce HIV acquisition using discreet methods such as topical biotherapeutics containing lactobacilli isolates that strongly suppress HIV infectivity that women can control themselves in order to improve their genital health. This infectivity assay may also be used to screen for the best lactobacilli isolates for use in biotherapeutics for HIV prevention in women.

CHAPTER 6: Immunomodulatory properties of cervicovaginal *Lactobacillus* isolates from South African women at high risk of HIV acquisition

6.1 Summary

Upregulated levels of FGT inflammatory cytokine responses increase HIV infection susceptibility in women. Non-optimal microbiota and BV which are characterised by depletion of *Lactobacillus* species and an overgrowth of facultative and strict anaerobic bacteria, are associated with increased FGT cytokine production. However, the microbial causes and the immunomodulatory effects of BV are not yet fully understood and effective treatment strategies do not exist. On the other hand, *Lactobacillus* species may protect against HIV partly by reducing inflammation in the FGT. The aim was to evaluate the immunoregulatory properties of vaginal lactobacilli, and determine the mechanisms underlying these relationships. A total of 80 lactobacilli isolates including *L. crispatus, L. jensenii, L. johnsonii, L. mucosae, L. plantarum, L. ruminis, L. salivarius, L. vaginalis* were isolated from South African women with non-optimal microbiota (n=18) and optimal microbiota (n=14). Production of nine cytokines by vaginal epithelial cells in response to lactobacilli, and two bacterial vaginosis-associated bacteria *Gardnerella vaginalis* ATCC 14018 and *P. bivia* ATCC 14018, was measured using Luminex. Adhesion to vaginal epithelial cells, growth rates, bacterial size, culture acidification and D/L-lactate production were evaluated. Lactobacilli from women with non-optimal microbiota produced less lactic acid and induced greater inflammatory cytokine production than those from women with optimal microbiota, with IL-6, IL-8, IL-1α, IL-1β, MIP-1α and MIP-1β production significantly elevated. Sixteen lactobacilli suppressed IL-6 and IL-8 responses to *G. vaginalis.* Interestingly, only *L. crispatus* isolates were able to markedly suppress cytokine responses to *P. bivia*, with significant decreases in IP-10, MIP-1α, MIP-1β, MIP-3α, IL-6, IL-1α and IL-8 concentration. Lactobacilli adhesion to epithelial cells correlated negatively with IL-6, IL-8, MIP-1α and IL-1RA production. *Lactobacillus* growth rates, bacterial sizes and adhesion to VK2 cells did not differ significantly between isolates from women with non-optimal microbiota versus those from women with optimal microbiota. These findings show that, while cervicovaginal lactobacilli resulted in reduced production of the majority of inflammatory cytokines in response to *G. vaginalis* and *P. bivia,* isolates from women with non-optimal microbiota were more inflammatory and produced less antimicrobial lactic acid than isolates from women with optimal microbiota.

6.2 Introduction

HIV remains a major public health concern, particularly in sub-Saharan Africa where young South African women are at an exceptionally high risk of becoming HIV-infected (UNAIDS, 2010; Harrison *et al.*, 2015). Increased production of inflammatory cytokines in the FGT increases HIV acquisition risk, likely by recruiting activated HIV target cells, such as CD4+ T-cells, to the vaginal mucosal epithelium, promoting HIV transcription via nuclear factor kappa B (NF-κB) activation, and reducing the integrity of the epithelial barrier (Arnold *et al.*, 2016; Doerflinger *et al.*, 2014; Klatt *et al.*, 2017; Osborn *et al.*, 1989; Anahtar *et al.*, 2015; Masson *et al.*, 2016). BV and non-optimal vaginal microbiota including *G. vaginalis, P. bivia, Atopobium* spp., *M. hominis* and *Mobiluncus* spp., are thought to be major drivers of FGT inflammation and HIV risk in sub-Saharan African women (Eastment *et al.*, 2015; Lennard *et al.*, 2017). BV also increases susceptibility to other STIs, including *C. trachomatis, N. gonorrhoeae* (Wiesenfeld *et al.*, 2003), *T. vaginalis* (Wiesenfeld *et al.*, 2003; Brotman *et al.*, 2010; Rathod *et al.*, 2012), human papillomavirus (Gillet *et al.*, 2011) and herpes simplex virus type 2 (HSV-2) (Cherpes *et al.*, 2003) and adverse reproductive health outcomes (Haggerty *et al.*, 2004; Ness *et al.*, 2005). Furthermore, HIV-infected women with BV are over 3-times more likely to transmit HIV to their partners (Cu-Uvin *et al.*, 2001; Cohen *et al.*, 2012). However, the pathogenesis and immunomodulatory effects of BV are not yet fully understood and current treatment strategies are only partially effective, with inflammatory cytokine concentrations remaining elevated even in women who are successfully treated (Bradshaw *et al.*, 2006; Joag *et al.*, 2018).

On the other hand, the normal vaginal microbiota of healthy pre-menopausal women is dominated by lactobacilli species, including *L. crispatus, L. jensenii, L. gasseri*, and *L. vaginalis* (Antonio *et al.*, 1999; Burton *et al.*, 2003; Anukam *et al.*, 2005; Fredricks *et al.*, 2005; Ravel *et al.*, 2011). *Lactobacillus* species appear to play a critical role in regulating inflammatory responses in the FGT and protecting against pathogens, including HIV (Anahtar *et al.*, 2015; Gosmann *et al.*, 2017). On the other hand, the role of *L. iners* is controversial as this species is associated with increased risk of conversion from an optimal to a non-optimal vaginal microbiome (Verstraelen *et al.*, 2009), acquisition of STIs (Van Houdt *et al.*, 2018) and upregulation of inflammatory responses (Doerflinger *et al.*, 2014).

The mechanisms underlying the protective properties of optimal *Lactobacillus* species are not fully understood, however it is thought that lactobacilli protect against pathogens by competitively excluding pathogen colonization, and producing antimicrobial compounds such as bacteriocins and lactic acid (Aroutcheva *et al.*, 2001; O'Hanlon *et al.*, 2011). Lactic acid exists as L- and D- isomers and it maintains a physiological pH of <4.5 in the FGT, which inhibits the growth of potential pathogens and may inactivate HIV virus particles (Aroutcheva *et al.*, 2001; Aldunate *et al.*, 2013; Tachedjian *et al.*, 2017). Competitive exclusion of pathogens may also modulate inflammation by preventing pathogen interaction with pattern recognition receptors (PRRs) present in the genital epithelium. Lactobacilli and the lactic acid that they produce may also downregulate inflammatory cytokine production by cervicovaginal epithelial cells, which may in turn reduce susceptibility to HIV (Hearps *et al.*, 2017; Chetwin *et al.*, 2019). A better understanding of the immunomodulatory and other properties of vaginal lactobacilli is critical for the development of biomedical interventions to improve BV treatment and reduce HIV infection risk in women. As few studies have characterised vaginal *Lactobacillus* isolates in African populations, the influence of optimal vaginal *Lactobacillus* species isolated from South African women, *G. vaginalis* ATCC 14018 and *P. bivia* ATCC 29303 on vaginal epithelial cell inflammatory responses was evaluated, as well as the possible underlying mechanisms.

6.3 Methods

Vaginal *Lactobacillus* isolates (n=80) including *L. crispatus*, *L. jensenii*, *L. johnsonii*, *L. mucosae*, *L. plantarum*, *L. ruminis*, *L. salivarius* and *L. vaginalis* were obtained from cervicovaginal secretions collected from young women who participated in the WISH study in Cape Town, South Africa. The isolates were cultured and stored as described in Chapter 2 and identified to species level using MALDI-TOF biotyping. Sixty-four of these isolates were used to stimulate VK2 cells in separate cultures, while the additional 16 isolates were used for pre-treatment of VK2 cells prior to stimulation with BV-associated bacteria. The 64 isolates were different from the 16 isolates analysed in Chapter 5 to further evaluate the finding that isolates obtained from women with BV were associated with greater inflammatory responses compared to isolates obtained from BV negative women, as observed in Chapters 4 and 5. The characteristics of the 64 *Lactobacillus* isolates are described in detail in Chapter 3. The characteristics of the additional 16 isolates are described in Chapter 5. Two BV-associated bacterial species (*G. vaginalis* ATCC 14018 and *P. bivia* ATCC 29303) obtained from ATCC were also analysed in this Chapter and the culture conditions are described in Chapter 2, section 2.5 and 2.6. The production of secreted interleukin (IL)-1α, IL-1β, IL-6, IL-8, IFN-γ-inducible protein (IP)-10, macrophage inflammatory protein (MIP)-1α, MIP-1β, MIP-3α and regulatory IL-1 receptor antagonist (RA) by vaginal epithelial cells in response to lactobacilli in the presence or absence of *G. vaginalis* ATCC 14018 and *P. bivia* ATCC 29303, was measured using Luminex as described in Chapter 2. Cytokine production was evaluated in VK2 cells and not in Ca Ski cells as VK2 cells would be more representative of the vaginal environment as these cells are obtained from vaginal tissue and are immortalized, rather than a cancer cell line.

6.4 Results

6.4.1 Study population and clinical *Lactobacillus* isolates

A total of 80 *Lactobacillus* isolates were obtained from the cervicovaginal secretions of 32 women who participated in the WISH study in Cape Town, South Africa [*L. crispatus* (n=15), *L. jensenii* (n=18), *L. johnsonii* (n=5), *L. mucosae* (n=19), *L. plantarum* (n=2), *L. ruminis* (n=5), *L. salivarius* (n=2), *L. vaginalis* (n=14)]. For this Chapter, 28 isolates were obtained from women with non-optimal [BV positive (n=28) and intermediate microbiota (n=8)] and 44 isolates from women with optimal microbiota (BV negative) (**Table 6.1**). The median age of the women was 18 (range 16-22) years and all of the women were taking hormonal contraceptives at the time of sample collection. Six of the women had *C. trachomatis* infections, three had *N. gonorrhoeae* infections, one had a *T. vaginalis* infection, one was shedding HSV-2 and only one participant was coinfected with *N. gonorrhoeae* and *C. trachomatis*. None of the participants tested positive for *T. pallidum* or had yeast infections.

Table 6.1. Demographic and clinical data of the study population

Clinical and laboratory findings	Optimal microbiota (N=14) n (%)	Non-optimal Microbiota (N=18) n (%)
Black race	14 (100)	18 (100)
Median age in years (range)	18.5 (16-20)	19 (16-22)
Chlamydia trachomatis (PCR positive)	3 (21)	3 (16.7)
Neisseria gonorrhoeae (PCR positive)	3 (21)	0 (0)
Trichomonas vaginalis (PCR positive)	1 (7)	0 (0)
Mycoplasma genitalium (PCR positive)	0 (0)	0 (0)
HSV-2 IgG positive	0 (0)	1 (5.6)
HSV (PCR positive)	0 (0)	0 (0)
Treponema pallidum (RPR>1:4, TPHA positive)	0 (0)	0 (0)
Yeast cells detected	0 (0)	0 (0)
PSA positive	1 (7)	8 (44.4)
Using DMPA	3 (21)	2 (11.1)
Using Nur-Isterate	10 (71)	12 (66.7)
Using Implanon	1 (7)	4 (22.2)

BV, bacterial vaginosis; PCR, polymerase chain reaction; HSV-2, herpes simplex virus type 2; RPR, rapid plasma reagin; TPHA, Treponema pallidum hemagglutination; PSA, prostate specific antigen; DMPA, depot medroxyprogesterone acetate

6.4.2 Production of inflammatory cytokines by VK2 cells in response to vaginal *Lactobacillus* isolates

Induction of cytokine production was highly varied between species. However, there were no significant differences in individual cytokines between species after adjusting for multiple comparisons and the level of within-species variation was high (**Figure 6.1**).

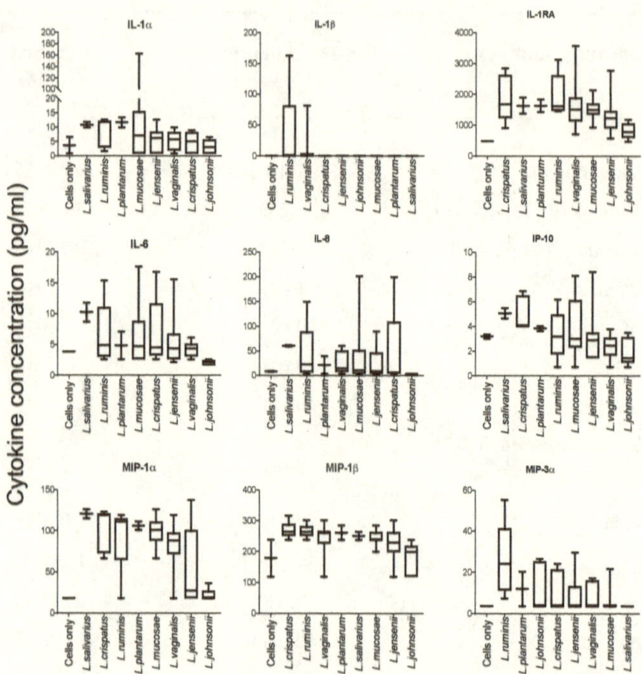

Figure 6.1: Cytokine production by vaginal epithelial cells (VK2) stimulated with clinical *Lactobacillus* isolates grouped according to species. VK2 cell monolayers were cultured to 80% confluency and then treated with *Lactobacillus* isolates including [*L. crispatus* (n=11), *L. jensenii* (n=14), *L. johnsonii* (n=5), *L. mucosae* (n=15), *L. plantarum* (n=2), *L. ruminis* (n=5), *L. salivarius* (n=2), *L. vaginalis* (n=10)] adjusted to 4.18x10^6 colony forming units (CFU)/ml before being incubated for 24 hours at 37°C with 5% CO_2. The concentrations of 9 cytokines were then measured in the culture supernatants using Luminex. Data are shown as box and whisker plots. Boxes represent the interquartile ranges, lines within boxes represent medians and whiskers represent minimum and maximum values. Adjusted p-values <0.05 were considered statistically significant.

Of the different species evaluated, *L. jensenii* and *L. johnsonii* isolates obtained from women with optimal microbiota tended to induce lower levels of cytokine production than the other lactobacilli species (**Figures 6.2 and 6.3**).

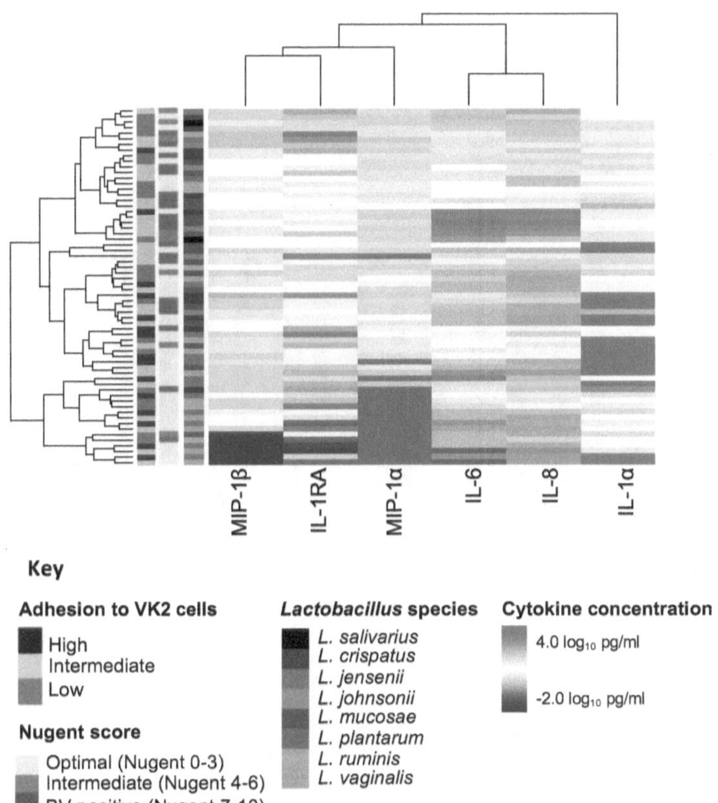

Figure 6.2: Heatmap of $\log_{10}$-transformed concentrations of cytokines produced by vaginal epithelial (VK2) cells in response to vaginal *Lactobacillus* isolates obtained from women with optimal (n=36 isolates) and non-optimal [intermediate (n=8 isolates) and bacterial vaginosis (n=20 isolates)]. VK2 cell monolayers were cultured to 80% confluency and then treated with *Lactobacillus* isolates including [*L. crispatus* (n=11), *L. jensenii* (n=14), *L. johnsonii* (n=5), *L. mucosae* (n=15), *L. plantarum* (n=2), *L. ruminis* (n=5), *L. salivarius* (n=2), *L. vaginalis* (n=10)] adjusted to 4.18×10^6 colony forming units (CFU)/ml before being incubated for 24 hours at 37°C with 5% CO_2. Cytokine concentrations in the cell culture supernatants were measured using Luminex.
The dendrogram above the heat map indicates relationships between the concentration profiles of the analyzed cytokines. The horizontal branches have arbitrary lengths and the lengths of the vertical branches indicate the degrees of similarity between the different cytokine profiles. Shorter branches indicate greater similarity, while longer ones indicate less similarity between cytokine profiles. The dendrogram on the left of the heatmap indicates relationships between the cytokine concentration profiles of the *Lactobacillus* isolates analysed. Shorter horizontal branch lengths between isolates reflect greater similarity between cytokines while longer branches show less similarity. Cytokine concentrations are indicated using a color scale that ranges from blue (low) through white to red (high). Level of adhesion to VK2 cells, BV status, and *Lactobacillus* species are also shown below the heatmap. Abbreviations: IL, interleukin; MIP, macrophage inflammatory protein; RA, receptor antagonist.

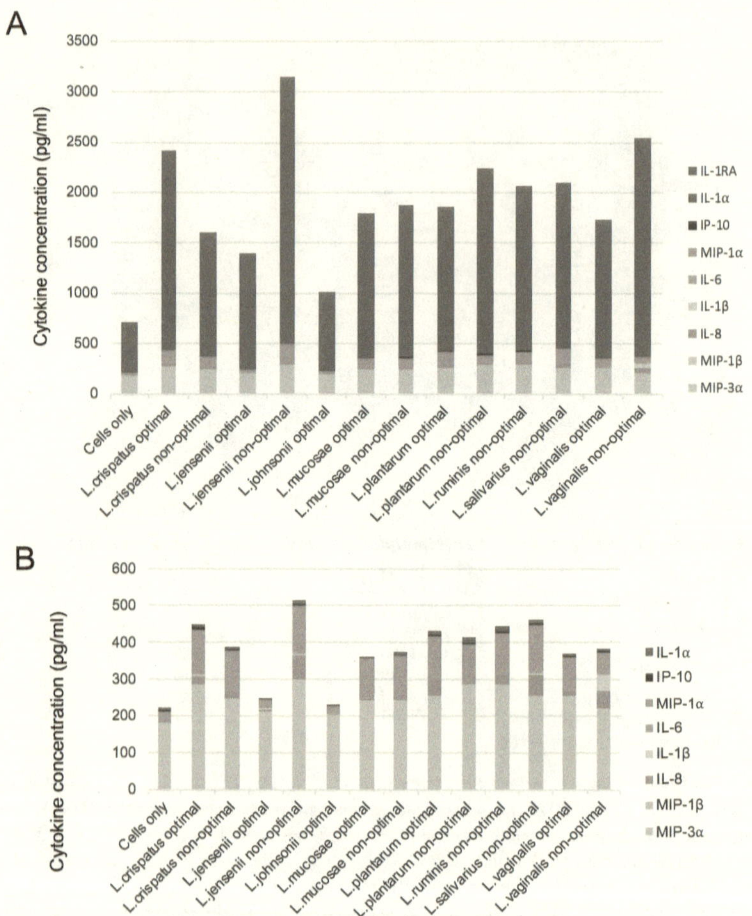

Figure 6.3: Inflammatory cytokine production by VK2 cells in response to different vaginal *Lactobacillus* species. Lactobacilli isolates including [*L. crispatus* (optimal n=6; non-optimal n=5), *L. jensenii* (optimal n=12; non-optimal n=2), *L. johnsonii* (optimal n=5), *L. mucosae* (optimal n=4; non-optimal n=11), *L. plantarum* (optimal n=1; non-optimal n=1), *L. ruminis* (non-optimal n=5), *L. salivarius* (non-optimal n=2), *L. vaginalis* (optimal n=8; non-optimal n=2)] were adjusted to 4.18×10^6 colony forming units (CFU)/ml in separate cultures before being incubated with VK2 cell monolayers at 80% confluency for 24 hours at 37°C with 5% CO_2. Cytokine concentrations were measured in the culture supernatants using Luminex. (**A**) Stacked bars showing cumulative median concentrations of each cytokine (IL-1α, IL-1β, IL-1RA, IL-6, IL-8, IP-10, MIP-1α, MIP-1β and MIP-3α) with the lactobacilli species stratified according to BV status (**B**) Stacked bars showing median concentrations of each pro-inflammatory cytokine (IL-1α, IL-1β, IL-6, IL-8, IP-10, MIP-1α, MIP-1β and MIP-3α), with anti-inflammatory IL-1RA excluded. Abbreviations: IL, interleukin; MIP, macrophage inflammatory protein; RA, receptor antagonist.

To determine whether inflammatory cytokine induction differed between lactobacilli obtained from women with optimal [BV negative (n=14)] and non-optimal [intermediate microbiota (n=5) and BV positive (n=13)] microbiota, vaginal epithelial (VK2) cells were stimulated with lactobacilli isolates and secreted pro-inflammatory cytokines (IL-6, IL-1α, IL-1β) chemokines (IL-8, IP-10, MIP-3α, MIP-1α, MIP-1β) and regulatory IL-1RA concentrations were measured in cell culture supernatants using Luminex. Lactobacilli obtained from women with intermediate microbiota or BV induced greater inflammatory responses than isolates from women with optimal microbiota (**Figure 6.4**). IL-6 [adjusted (adj.) p=0.020], IL-8 (adj. p=0.011), IL-1α (adj. p=0.020), MIP-1α (adj. p=0.020), MIP-1β (adj. p=0.040) and IL-1RA (adj. p=0.030) production in response to isolates from women with non-optimal was significantly greater than lactobacilli from women with optimal microbiota (**Figure 6.4**).

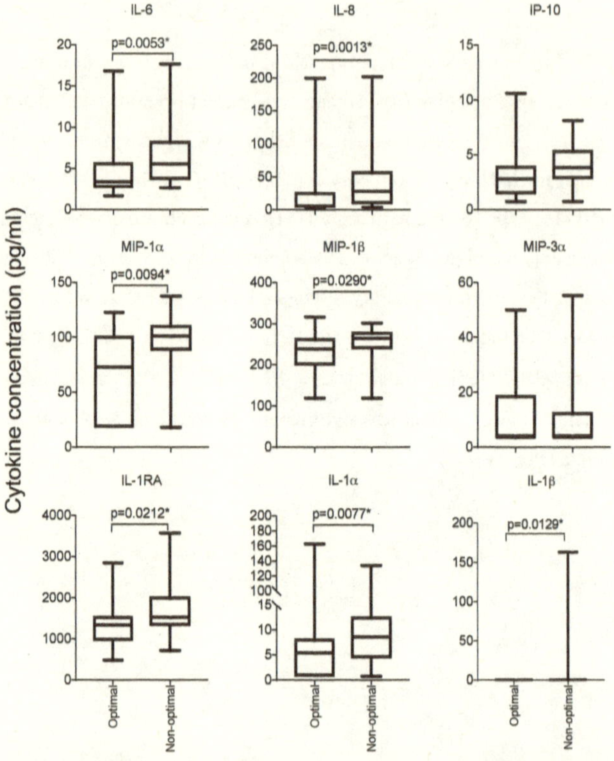

Figure 6.4: Inflammatory cytokine production in response to *Lactobacillus* isolates from women with optimal microbiota (n=36 isolates; Nugent 0-3) compared to women with non-optimal microbiota (Nugent 4-10; n=20 isolates). *Lactobacillus* cultures including [*L. crispatus* (n=6); *L. jensenii* (n=12), *L. johnsonii* (n=5), *L. mucosae* (n=4), *L. plantarum* (n=1), *L. vaginalis* (n=8)] compared to women with dysbiosis (Nugent 4-10; n=28) including [*L. crispatus* (n=5), *L. jensenii* (n=2), *L. mucosae* (n=11), *L. plantarum* (n=1), *L. ruminis* (n=5), *L. salivarius* (n=2) and *L. vaginalis* (n=2)] were adjusted to 4.18x10^6 colony forming units (CFU)/ml then added to VK2 cell monolayers at 80% confluency before being incubated for 24 hours at 37°C with 5% CO_2. Cytokine concentrations in the cell culture supernatants were measured using Luminex. Data are shown as Tukey box plots. Boxes represent the interquartile ranges, lines within boxes represent medians and whiskers represent minimum and maximum values. P-values were adjusted for multiple comparisons using a false discovery rate step down procedure. *Adjusted p-values <0.05 were considered statistically significant.

Similar responses were observed when evaluating inflammatory responses induced by isolates from women with intermediate microbiota and BV separately (**Figure 6.5**).

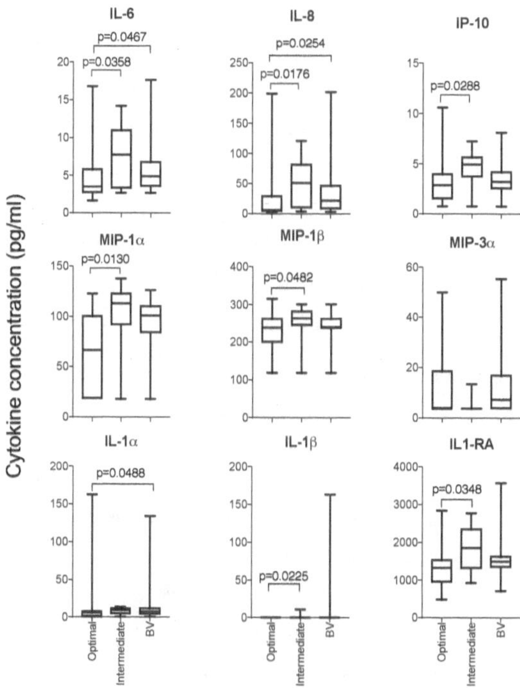

Figure 6.5: Cytokine production by vaginal epithelial (VK2) cells in response to vaginal *Lactobacillus* isolates. *Lactobacillus* isolates (n=64) obtained from women with optimal (n=36 isolates), non-optimal [intermediate (n=8 isolates) and bacterial vaginosis (BV) (n=20 isolates)] were cultured and adjusted to 4.18×10^6 colony forming units (CFU)/ml in antibiotic free keratinocyte serum free media then added to VK2 cell monolayers at 80% confluency before being incubated for 24 hours at 37°C with 5% CO_2. Cytokine concentrations in the cell culture supernatants were measured using Luminex. Data are shown as Tukey box plots. Boxes represent the interquartile ranges, lines within boxes represent medians and whiskers represent minimum and maximum values. P-values were adjusted for multiple comparisons using a false discovery rate step down procedure. *Adjusted p-values <0.05 were considered statistically significant.

Logistic regression was used to evaluate the relationship between inflammatory responses to the *Lactobacillus* isolates and the BV status of the women, adjusting for possible confounders, including the presence of semen which may contain lactobacilli (Weng *et al.*, 2014), the use of contraceptives that may influence the microbial populations present (Brooks *et al.*, 2017) and STIs which are associated with BV status (Rathod *et al.*, 2012; Wiesenfeld *et al.*, 2003). The relationships between BV status and IL-6 [β-coefficient: 2.71; 95% confidence interval (CI): 0.40-

5.01; p=0.021], IL-8 (β-coefficient: 1.44; 95% CI: 0.34-2.53; p=0.010), MIP-1α (β-coefficient: 1.83; 95% CI: 0.06-3.60; p=0.043) and IL-1RA (β-coefficient: 4.00; 95% CI: 0.39-7.62; p=0.030) remained significant after adjusting for *Lactobacillus* species, semen contamination [determined by prostate specific antigen (PSA) measurement in the cervicovaginal secretions] and contraceptive use during the time of sample collection. Following adjustment for STI status, MIP-1α (β-coefficient: 1.90; 95% CI: 0.11-3.70; p=0.038) and IL-8 (β-coefficient: 1.21; 95% CI: 0.13-2.29; p=0.028) remained significantly associated with BV status.

6.4.3 Production of inflammatory cytokines by VK2 cells in response to *G. vaginalis* in the presence and absence of vaginal *Lactobacillus* isolates

Previous studies have suggested that *Lactobacillus* species and their metabolites may suppress inflammatory responses to vaginal pathogens and pathobionts (Hearps *et al.*, 2017; Chetwin *et al.*, 2019). To investigate this, inflammatory cytokine production by VK2 cells in response to *G. vaginalis* was evaluated. Stimulating the cells with *G. vaginalis* induced production of IL-8 (adj. p=0.005), IL-6 (adj. p=0.005), MIP-1α (adj. p=0.014), MIP-1β (adj. p=0.005), MIP-3α (adj. p=0.005) and IL-1α (adj. p=0.005). Pretreating the cells with lactobacilli suppressed production of IL-6 (adj. p=0.002) and IL-8 (adj. p=0.024) in response to *G. vaginalis,* while non-significant decreases in MIP-1α, MIP-1β, and MIP-3α were observed (**Figure 6.6A**). However, pre-incubation with lactobacilli prior to *G. vaginalis* stimulation significantly increased the production of IL-1α (adj. p=0.010) and IL-1β (adj. p=0.002) relative to *G. vaginalis* alone. Overall, *L. jensenii* isolates suppressed cytokine responses to *G. vaginalis* to the greatest degree, followed by *L. crispatus, L. vaginalis* and *L. mucosae* (**Figure 6.6B**). A viability assay was carried out in order to investigate whether the bacterial stimulation assays were not causing cell death. The cells were treated with the bacteria for the same period of time as in the cytokine stimulation assays before using the trypan blue exclusion method to determine cell viability. The bacterial stimulations showed no evidence of cytotoxicity to the VK2 cells after bacterial stimulations (**Figure 6.7**).

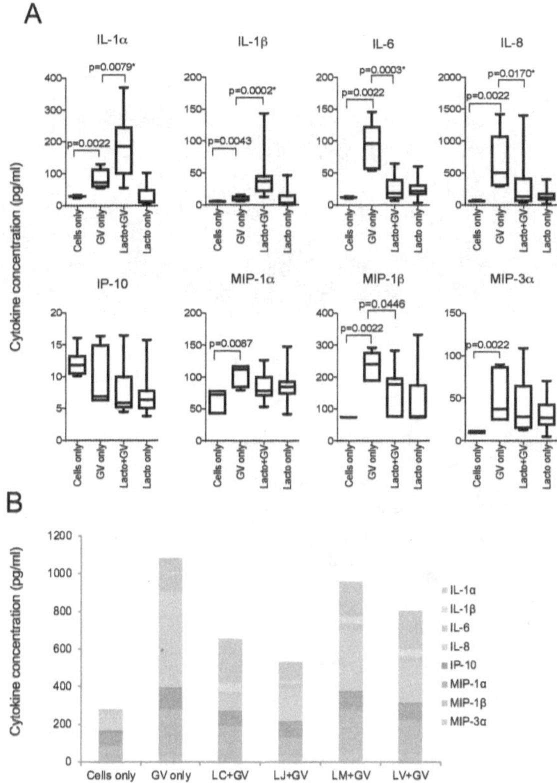

Figure 6.6: Cytokine production by VK2 cells in response to *Gardnerella vaginalis* in the presence or absence of clinical *Lactobacillus* isolates (n=16). VK2 cells were cultured to 80% confluency and then each well was treated with a single *Lactobacillus* species including [*L. crispatus* (n=4); *L. jensenii* (n=4); *L. mucosae* (n=4) and *L. vaginalis* (n=4)] adjusted to 4.18x10^6 colony forming units (CFU)/ml before being incubated for 5 hours at 37°C with 5% CO_2. *G. vaginalis* cultures at a concentration of 1x10^7 CFU/ml were then added and incubated for a further 20 hours. Cytokine concentrations were measured in duplicates in the culture supernatants using Luminex. (**A**) Data are presented as Tukey box plots. Boxes represent the interquartile ranges, lines within boxes represent medians and whiskers represent minimum and maximum values. Mann Whitney U tests were used to compare cytokine responses and p-values were adjusted for multiple comparisons using a false discovery rate step down procedure. *Adjusted p-values <0.05 were considered to be statistically significant. (**B**) Stacked bars showing the median concentrations of all pro-inflammatory cytokines produced by VK2 cells in response to *G. vaginalis* in the presence or absence of different clinical *Lactobacillus* species. LC, *Lactobacillus crispatus*; LJ, *Lactobacillus jensenii*; LM, *Lactobacillus mucosae*; LV, *Lactobacillus vaginalis*

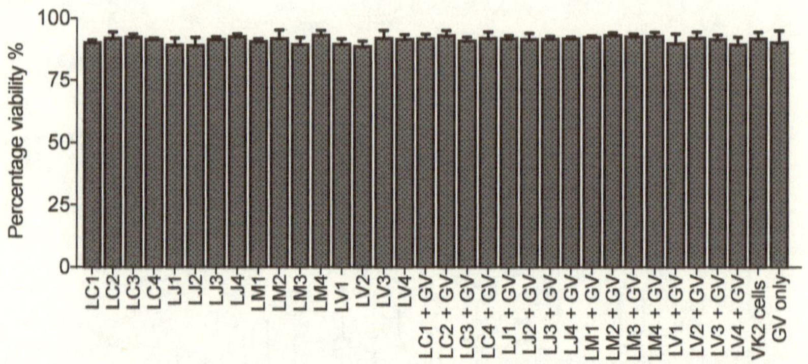

Figure 6.7: Vaginal epithelial cells (VK2) cell viability following bacterial stimulation. VK2 cells were cultured to 80% confluency and then treated with *Lactobacillus* isolates adjusted to 4.18x10^6 colony forming units (CFU)/ml in antibiotic free keratinocyte serum free media (KSFM) before being incubated for 5 hours at 37°C with 5% CO_2. *G. vaginalis* cultures at a concentration of 1x10^7 CFU/ml were then added and cultures were incubated for a further 20 hours. The bars show the percentage of viable cells in relation to the total number of cells and correspond to the mean ± standard deviation of the experiments that were performed in triplicate. LC, *Lactobacillus crispatus*; LJ, *Lactobacillus jensenii*; LM, *Lactobacillus mucosae*; LV, *Lactobacillus vaginalis*

6.4.4 Vaginal epithelial cell inflammatory responses to *P. bivia* in the presence and absence of vaginal *Lactobacillus* isolates

To investigate whether the vaginal *Lactobacillus* isolates had a similar effect on inflammatory responses to *P. bivia* compared to *G. vaginalis*, inflammatory cytokine production by VK2 cells in responses to *P. bivia* were evaluated. Stimulation of the VK2 cells with *P. bivia* caused non-significant increases in IP-10, MIP-1α, MIP-1β, MIP-3α, IL-6, IL-1α and IL-8 production. Pretreatment of the cells with *L. crispatus* reduced production of IP-10 (adj. p=0.048), MIP-1α (adj. p=0.045), MIP-1β (adj. p=0.048), MIP-3α (adj. p=0.048), IL-6 (adj. p=0.048), IL-1α (p=0.048). However, IL-8 (p=0.0121) suppression did not remain significant after adjusting for multiple comparisons (**Figure 6.8A**). Significant suppression of IP-10 responses were also observed when the cells were pretreated with *L. jensenii* (p=0.012) and *L. mucosae* (p=0.012) isolates but did not remain significant after adjusting for multiple comparisons (**Figure 6.8A**).

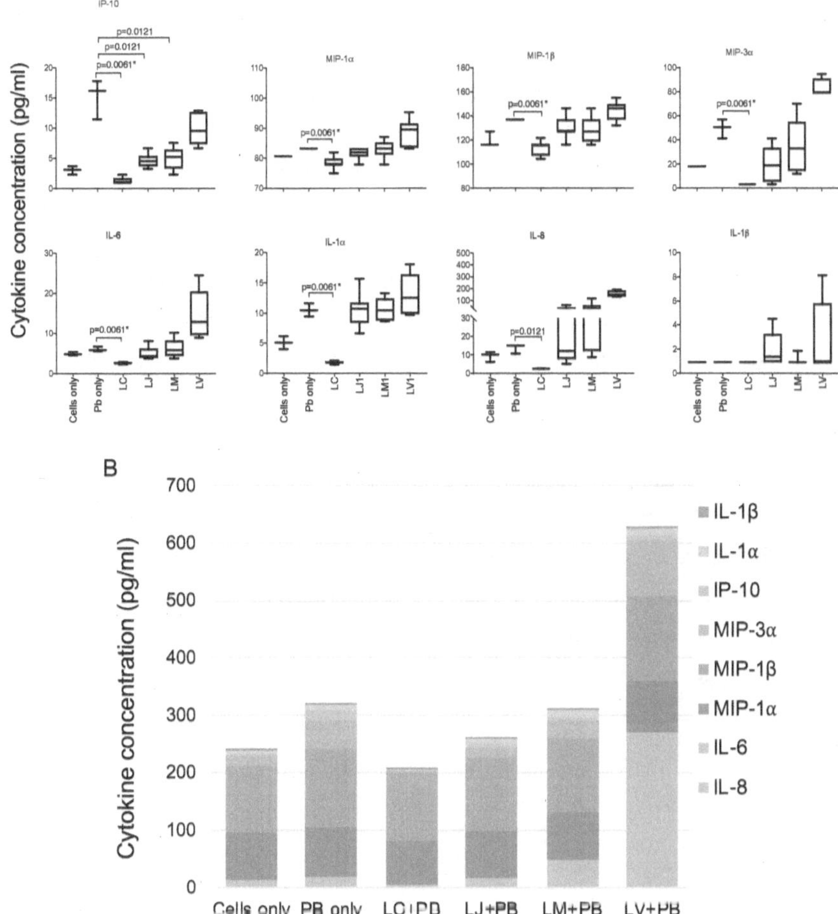

Figure 6.8: Cytokine production by VK2 cells in response to *Prevotella bivia* in the presence or absence of clinical *Lactobacillus* isolates (n=16). VK2 cell monolayers were cultured to 80% confluency and then treated with *Lactobacillus* isolates including [*L. crispatus* (n=4); *L. jensenii* (n=4); *L. mucosae* (n=4) and *L. vaginalis* (n=4)] adjusted to 4.18×10^6 colony forming units (CFU)/ml in separate cultures before being incubated for 5 hours at 37°C with 5% CO_2. *P. bivia* cultures at a concentration of 1×10^9 CFU/ml were then added and incubated for a further 20 hours. Cytokine concentrations were measured in duplicate in the culture supernatants using Luminex. (**A**) Data are presented as Tukey box plots. Boxes represent the interquartile ranges, lines within boxes represent medians and whiskers represent minimum and maximum values. Mann Whitney U tests were used to compare cytokine responses and p-values were adjusted for multiple comparisons using a false discovery rate step down procedure. *Adjusted p-values <0.05 were considered to be statistically significant. (**B**) Stacked bars showing the cumulative median concentrations of all inflammatory cytokines produced by VK2 cells in response to *P. bivia* in the presence or absence of different vaginal *Lactobacillus* species. PB, *Prevotella bivia;* LC, *Lactobacillus crispatus*; LJ, *Lactobacillus jensenii*; LM, *Lactobacillus mucosae*; LV, *Lactobacillus vaginalis.*

6.4.5 Influence of *Lactobacillus* adhesion to vaginal epithelial cells and D-lactate concentration on production of inflammatory cytokines

As lactic acid production by lactobacilli, as well as competitive exclusion of pathogens, may influence inflammatory responses, the relationships between inflammatory cytokines and lactate production and adhesion to vaginal epithelial cells were next evaluated. Overall, highly adherent isolates induced lower cytokine responses (**Figure 6.2**). *Lactobacillus* adhesion to VK2 cells correlated negatively with IL-6 (p=0.0018, adj. p=0.0162, rho=-0.3835), IL-8 (p=0.0242, adj. p=0.0726, rho=-0.2815), MIP-1α (p=0.0233, adj. p=0.0726, rho=-0.2833) and IL-1RA (p=0.0355, adj. p=0.080 rho=-0.2633).

To further investigate the impact of competitive binding of the lactobacilli to the VK2 cells, a variation of the cytokine assay was carried out in which unbound lactobacilli were then washed off with PBS before *G. vaginalis* was added. It was found that washing off unbound lactobacilli reduced the level of inflammatory cytokine suppression (**Figure 6.9**), suggesting that the unbound lactobacilli also contribute to the immunoregulatory effect, perhaps through the production of metabolites such as lactic acid.

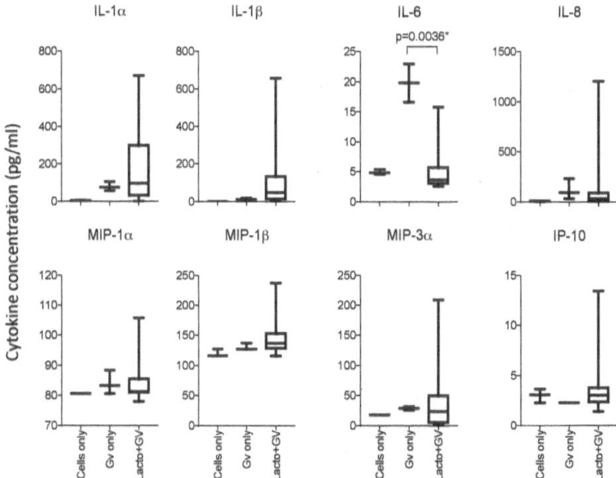

Figure 6.9: Cytokine production by vaginal epithelial (VK2) cells in response to *G. vaginalis* in the presence or absence of clinical *Lactobacillus* isolates. VK2 cell monolayers were cultured to 80% confluency and then treated with *Lactobacillus* isolates including [*L. crispatus* (n=4); *L. jensenii* (n=4); *L. mucosae* (n=4) and *L. vaginalis* (n=4)] adjusted to 4.18×10^6 colony forming units (CFU)/ml before being incubated for 5 hours at 37°C with 5% CO_2. Cells were washed three times with sterile PBS to remove unbound lactobacilli before *G. vaginalis* cultures at a concentration of 1×10^7 CFU/ml were added and incubated for a further 20 hours. Data are presented as Tukey box plots. Boxes represent the interquartile ranges, lines within boxes represent medians and whiskers represent minimum and maximum values. Mann Whitney U tests were used to compare cytokine responses and p-values were adjusted for multiple comparisons using a false discovery rate step down procedure. *Adjusted p-values <0.05 were considered to be statistically significant.

While L-lactate, culture pH, average bacterial length and growth rates were not associated with cytokine production, D-lactate production was negatively correlated with IL-6 concentrations in *Lactobacillus/G. vaginalis* co-cultures (rho=-0.6269; p=0.0082; adj. p=0.066) (**Figure 6.10A**), although this association was not upheld after adjusting for multiple comparisons. A negative trend towards an association between D-lactate and IL-8 production was also observed in these co-cultures (rho=-0.4971; p=0.0501) (**Figure 6.10B**). There was no correlation between lactate concentration and cytokine production in the *Lactobacillus/P. bivia* co-cultures. Together these findings suggest that both D-lactate production and the direct interaction between the lactobacilli and epithelial cells may play an important role in regulation of inflammatory responses by the lactobacilli.

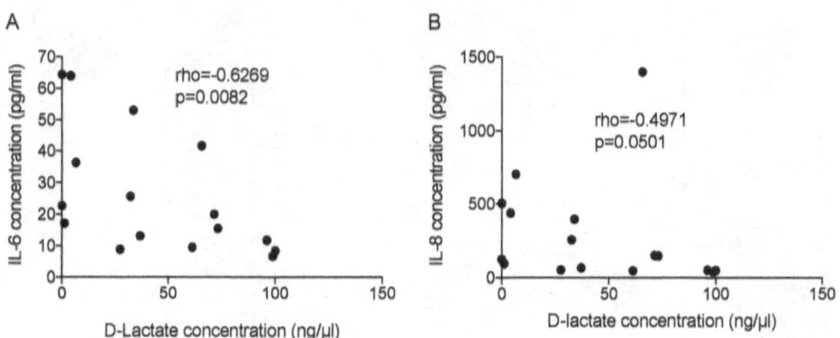

Figure 6.10: Spearman correlations between D-lactate concentration and IL-6 and IL-8 concentrations. VK2 cell monolayers were cultured to 80% confluency and then treated with vaginal *Lactobacillus* isolates adjusted to 4.18×10^6 colony forming units (CFU)/ml before being incubated for 5 hours at 37°C with 5% CO_2. *G. vaginalis* cultures at a concentration of 1×10^7 CFU/ml were then added and incubated for a further 20 hours. Supernatants were collected and the concentrations of D-lactate and L-lactate were determined by ELISA assays. P-values <0.05 were considered to be statistically significant.

6.4.6 Association between inflammatory responses and HIV pseudovirus infectivity

To determine whether the abilities of the isolates to induce inflammatory responses were related to their impact on HIV infectivity, associations between inflammatory cytokine production by VK2 cells stimulated with lactobacilli for 25 hours and the reduction in HIV infectivity by lactobacilli culture supernatants were evaluated. Interestingly, HIV infectivity correlated positively with IL-1α (rho=0.6210; p=0.01) and IL-1β (rho=0.6539; p=0.006) production by VK2 cells incubated with the same isolates (**Figure 6.11**).

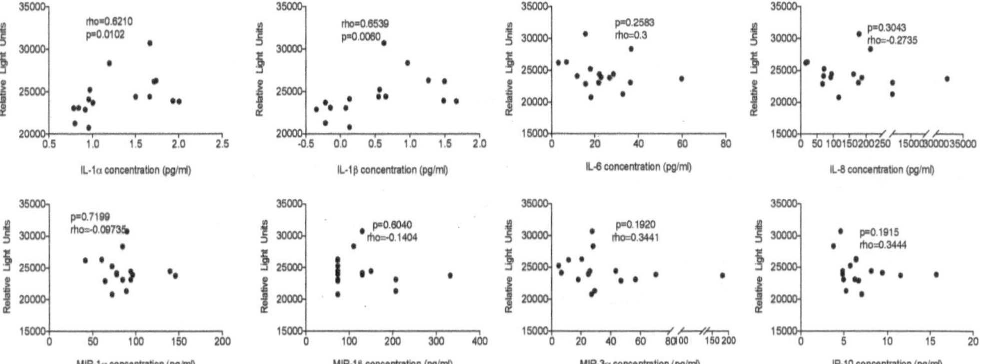

Figure 6.11: Spearman correlations between HIV pseudovirus entry and inflammatory cytokine concentrations. (**A**) Correlation between pseudovirus entry, IL-1α, IL-1β, I-6, IL-8, MIP-1α, MIP-1β, MIP-3α and IP-10 concentrations. VK2 cell monolayers were cultured to 80% confluency and then treated with vaginal *Lactobacillus* isolates adjusted to 4.18×10^6 colony forming units (CFU)/ml before being incubated for 24 hours at 37°C with 5% CO_2. Cytokine concentrations were measured in duplicate in the culture supernatants using Luminex. TZM-bl cells were seeded at 1×10^4 cells/well in a 96 well tissue culture plate and incubated at 37°C with 5% CO_2 for 24 hours. 50 µl of HIV pseudovirus was added in triplicate to the TZM-bl cells and incubated at 37°C with 5% CO_2 with 10µl of conditioned culture medium from lactobacilli including [*L. crispatus* (n=4), *L. jensenii* (n=4), *L. mucosae* (n=4) and *L. vaginalis* (n=4)] with a pseudovirus-only control well. P-values <0.05 were considered to be statistically significant.

6.5 Discussion

Understanding the characteristics of *Lactobacillus* species and strains that may influence genital tract inflammatory cytokine responses and pathogen colonization is critical for the development of more effective treatment strategies for BV in order to move the field of HIV prevention in young women forward. In this Chapter, *in vitro* systems were used to measure the concentrations of proinflammatory cytokines secreted by vaginal epithelial cells in response to 80 optimal vaginal *Lactobacillus* isolates and *G. vaginalis* and *P. bivia*, key BV-associated bacterial species. It was found that *Lactobacillus* isolates from women with non-optimal microbiota (Nugent score: 4-10) were significantly more inflammatory than isolates from women with optimal microbiota (Nugent score: 0-3). It was further found that a subset of 16 *Lactobacillus* isolates was able to significantly suppress inflammatory responses to *G. vaginalis,* while *L. crispatus* isolates were able to suppress inflammatory responses to *P. bivia* and *L. jensenii* and *L. mucosae* isolates suppressed IP-10 production. *Lactobacillus* isolates that induced greater inflammatory responses produced less D-lactate than those that induced little inflammatory cytokine production by VK2 cells. Additionally, less adherent lactobacilli were more inflammatory than those that strongly adhered to vaginal epithelial cells.

Here, a large variation was observed in the inflammatory properties of vaginal *Lactobacillus* strains, even those of the same species. This highlights the need to understand not just species level changes, but also strain level variation in microbiome studies. Previous studies have shown that women with non-optimal microbiota have higher levels of genital inflammation compared to women with *Lactobacillus*-dominant microbiota (Anahtar *et al.*, 2015; Lennard *et al.*, 2017). However, to the best of the author's knowledge, no other study has compared the properties of lactobacilli isolated from women with non-optimal microbiota to those of women with optimal microbiota. These findings suggest that the lactobacilli themselves may contribute to the inflammatory profile associated with FGT non-optimal microbiota, although, given the low relative abundance of lactobacilli in women with non-optimal microbiota (Ravel *et al.*, 2011; Anahtar *et al.*, 2015; Lennard *et al.*, 2017), this contribution may be minimal.

Although some lactobacilli induced inflammatory responses when cultured with vaginal epithelial cells in isolation, overall the lactobacilli significantly suppressed inflammatory responses to *G.*

vaginalis, while some suppressed responses to *P. bivia*. In this Chapter, incubation of vaginal epithelial cells with *G. vaginalis* alone caused significant upregulation of multiple inflammatory cytokines (IL-6, IL-8, IL-1α, MIP-1α, MIP-1β and MIP-3α), while pre-incubation with lactobacilli resulted in significant downregulation of IL-6 and IL-8 and nonsignificant downregulation of each of the chemokines evaluated. These findings are similar to previous studies showing that *G. vaginalis* induces inflammatory responses both *in vitro* and *in vivo* and lactobacilli have immunoregulatory properties *in vitro* and are associated with low inflammatory cytokine levels *in vivo* (Rose *et al.*, 2012; Santos *et al.*, 2018; Chetwin *et al.*, 2019). Although the majority of inflammatory cytokines and chemokines were lower following pre-incubation with lactobacilli, it was found that IL-1α and IL-1β production was significantly higher. This suggests that co-culture of vaginal epithelial cells with both lactobacilli and *G. vaginalis* had an additive effect on the IL-1 pathway and that the production of the other cytokines assessed may be regulated through alternative pathways. Furthermore, the IL-1 pathway is regulated both post-transcriptionally and translationally and involves more complex regulated checkpoints compared to other cytokine systems (Carta *et al.*, 2013; Mayer-Barber & Yan, 2017), which may explain the difference in expression of IL-1 compared to other cytokines observed here. Nevertheless, the fact that the majority of cytokines were suppressed by lactobacilli and cumulative median cytokine levels were lower following pre-incubation with lactobacilli compared to *G. vaginalis* only cultures suggests that lactobacilli may decrease HIV acquisition risk by reducing inflammatory cytokine production in the FGT. The mechanisms by which *G. vaginalis* induces inflammatory responses are not fully understood, however studies have shown that *G. vaginalis* produces a toxin, vaginolysin, that is cytolytic to host cells (Gelber *et al.*, 2008). Damaged tissue releases danger associated molecular patterns which activate pattern recognition receptors to induce a pro-inflammatory response (Tang *et al.*, 2012). It has further been reported that vaginolysin treatment of HeLa cells *in vitro* activates the p38 mitogen activated protein kinase pathway and increases IL-8 production (Gelber *et al.*, 2008). Recently it has been shown that *L. crispatus* is able to suppress vaginolysin expression by *G. vaginalis* (Castro *et al.*, 2018), providing a possible mechanism for the reduced production of some of the cytokines observed in this Chapter.

Incubation with *P. bivia* caused significant upregulation of IP-10 and non-significant upregulation of MIP-1α, MIP-1β, MIP-3α, IL-6, IL-1α and IL-8, as previously shown (Doerflinger *et al.*, 2014).

Interestingly, only *L. crispatus* isolates were able to markedly suppress cytokine production, with significant decreases in IP-10, MIP-1α, MIP-1β, MIP-3α, IL-6, IL-1α and IL-8 concentration. On the other hand, only IP-10 responses were significantly suppressed when the cells were pretreated with *L. jensenii* and *L. mucosae* isolates. A previous study showed that co-culturing *P. bivia* with vaginal lactobacilli reduced the viability of *P. bivia* with varying levels of efficacy between species (Atassi *et al*., 2006), which may explain the variation in level of suppression observed between the different lactobacilli species in this Chapter. It is not clear why stimulation with *P. bivia* cultures only caused mostly non-significant increases in cytokine production, as this species has been associated with high levels of inflammation *in vivo* (Jousimies–Somer, 1997; Hummelen *et al*., 2010). It is possible that the *P. bivia* strain used here is less inflammatory than others, or alternatively *P. bivia* isolates may possess mechanisms to evade host defense factors in order to establish an infection (Strömbeck *et al*., 2007). This finding suggests that commensals and pathogens may not be as distinct regarding inflammatory profiles (Doerflinger *et al*., 2014).

In order to identify possible underlying mechanisms for the increased inflammatory response to lactobacilli from women with non-optimal microbiota that was observed, a range of properties of the lactobacilli that may influence inflammatory cytokine induction, including D-lactate, L-lactate and lactic acid production, culture acidification, growth rates, adhesion to vaginal epithelial cells and *Lactobacillus* sizes were evaluated. D-lactate production by *Lactobacillus* isolates was inversely associated with cytokine production in the *Lactobacillus/G.vaginalis* co-cultures, supporting the results of previous studies demonstrating that lactic acid can have anti-inflammatory effects *in vitro* (Hearps *et al*., 2017). However, there was no correlation between lactate production and cytokine responses to *P. bivia.* Additionally, adhesion of lactobacilli to vaginal epithelial cells was inversely associated with cytokine responses, suggesting that direct interaction between the isolates and vaginal epithelial cells is critical for immunoregulation. Previous studies have suggested that the peptidoglycan cell wall, the proteins present in the cell wall, as well as the cell membrane, may influence the immunomodulatory properties of *Lactobacillus* species (Kulakauskas and Chapot-Chartier, 2014). Thus, differential adhesion capabilities may reflect differences in cell wall and membrane properties. It was found that removing unbound lactobacilli and the culture supernatant prior to addition of *G. vaginalis* reduced the level of suppression of inflammatory responses, although cytokine downregulation was still observed. The reduction in cytokine secretion observed in the *Lactobacillus/G.vaginalis* co-cultures may thus be due to competitive exclusion of *G. vaginalis* interaction with the vaginal epithelial cells as well as an effect of metabolites being secreted by the lactobacilli. It has been shown previously that lactobacilli were able to reduce *G. vaginalis* adhesion to the mucosal epithelium by approximately 60% (Cribby *et al.*, 2008) and that *G. vaginalis* was displaced from vaginal cells by lactobacilli (Boris *et al.*, 1998). Previous studies have additionally shown that vaginal lactobacilli reduce the expression of toll-like receptor (TLR)-4, which recognizes lipopolysaccharide (LPS) in the cell walls of gram negative bacteria (Zariffard *et al.*, 2005; Janssens and Beyaert, 2003; Tobita *et al.*, 2016). This suggests that lactobacilli may suppress immune responses at the level of pathogen recognition. Additionally, studies using cell lines have found that lactobacilli interfere with the nuclear factor kappa light-chain-enhancer of activated B cells (NF-kB) pathway, reducing inflammatory responses *in vitro* (Kim *et al.*, 2006; Lee *et al.*, 2008; Karlsson *et al.*, 2012).

HIV infectivity was also associated with IL-1α, as well as IL-1β production by VK2 cells in response to the same isolates. IL-1 is associated with activation of NF-Kβ which promotes HIV viral replication (Muzio *et al.*, 1998; Osborn *et al.*, 1989; Wira *et al.*, 2005), suggesting that an upregulation of these cytokines in the FGT may increase HIV acquisition risk as has previously been reported (Nazli *et al.*, 2010; Osborn *et al.*, 1989; Wira *et al.*, 2005). However, a limitation of this study was that HIV pseudovirus entry was tested in TZM-bl cells *in vitro* and not in the actual vaginal epithelial cells in which cytokine responses were evaluated.

Although these findings provide valuable information about the inflammatory properties of clinical *Lactobacillus* species and strains, a limitation is that an *in vitro* model including a transformed primary cell line was utilized to evaluate the characteristics of *Lactobacillus* isolates and this environment does not perfectly mimic *in vivo* conditions. Another limitation is that we were not powered to examine differences in the inflammatory nature within individual species.

In summary, these data show that non-*iners* vaginal *Lactobacillus* isolates induce varying levels of inflammatory cytokine production when cultured with vaginal epithelial cells, while isolates from women with non-optimal microbiota were more inflammatory *in vitro* than isolates from women with optimal microbiota. However, pre-incubation of vaginal epithelial cells with lactobacilli prior to the addition of *G. vaginalis*, resulted in decreases in the majority of the cytokines assessed. These findings suggest that the properties of the particular *Lactobacillus* strains present in the FGT (including lactic acid production and inflammatory nature) may influence the ability of non-optimal bacteria to colonize this compartment and shows that the immunomodulatory mechanisms of lactobacilli are multifactorial. This is relevant to biotherapeutic development, suggesting that it is critical to obtain *Lactobacillus* isolates from women with optimal microbiota and to fully characterise the inflammatory properties of potential vaginal probiotics.

CHAPTER 7: Comparative analysis of differentially abundant proteins in vaginal *Lactobacillus* isolates according to inflammatory profiles

7.1 Summary

Lactobacilli were found to suppress inflammatory responses in this and previous studies, however the immunomodulatory properties of individual *Lactobacillus* strains were found to be highly diverse, as described in Chapter 6. Inflammatory cytokine production by VK2 cells in response to the isolates was linked to D-lactate production, however this association was only significant for IL-6. To further understand the characteristics of the lactobacilli that may explain the varying inflammatory properties, mass spectrometry was used to compare overall protein expression between non-inflammatory and relatively inflammatory isolates. Total protein was extracted from 44 lactobacilli isolates including 8 species (*L. crispatus, L. jensenii, L. johnsonii, L. mucosae, L. plantarum, L. ruminis, L. salivarius* and *L. vaginalis*), of which 22 induced low levels and 22 induced high levels of cytokine production by VK2 cells. Liquid chromatography tandem mass spectrometry (LC-MS/MS) analysis was conducted with a Q-Exactive quadrupole-Orbitrap MS. Raw files were processed with MaxQuant version 1.5.7.4 against a database including the *Lactobacillus* genus and common contaminants. A total of 5087 proteins were identified and of these, 164 proteins were differentially abundant between the non-inflammatory and inflammatory lactobacilli isolates. The majority of the differentially abundant proteins (147/164) were assigned to *L. jensenii* and *L. johnsonii* species. Functional analysis revealed that 3/6 of the cellular components that were underabundant in inflammatory isolates were membrane-associated. The majority of the molecular functions that were underabundant in inflammatory isolates were enzymatic pathways, suggesting that less inflammatory isolates had greater metabolic activity. Surface protein aggregation promoting factor correlated positively with the level of adhesion to VK2 cells, although this was not upheld after adjusting for species and batch number. Ribonucleoside-triphosphate reductase enzyme and UPF0342 protein LRC_11170 were differentially abundant between lactobacilli that were highly adherent versus isolates with lower adhesion levels. D-lactate production was positively correlated with D-lactate dehydrogenase relative abundance and D-lactate dehydrogenase was strongly inversely associated with inflammatory cytokine responses. These findings show that the differences in inflammatory properties observed between lactobacilli strains may be associated with differences in proteome profiles of the isolates.

7.2 Introduction

The microenvironment of the FGT serves as a niche for a vast number of microorganisms that express diverse functional genes (Berard *et al*., 2018). A *Lactobacillus*-dominated microbiota with a low bacterial diversity is considered to be beneficial and protective against STIs, non-optimal microbiota and adverse reproductive health outcomes in women (Anahtar *et al*., 2015; Gosmann *et al*., 2017; Van De Wijgert *et al*., 2014). *Lactobacillus* species also appear to play a critical role in regulating inflammatory responses in the FGT, however the mechanisms underlying these properties are not fully understood (Anahtar *et al*., 2015; Gosmann *et al*., 2017; Chetwin *et al*., 2019). It has been suggested that the peptidoglycan cell wall, cell wall proteins, as well as the cell membrane, may influence the immunomodulatory properties of *Lactobacillus* species (Kulakauskas & Chapot-Chartier, 2014). The cell wall also maintains the bacterial cell integrity and mediates interactions between the bacteria and host cells (Kulakauskas & Chapot-Chartier, 2014). Additionally, it has also been shown that lactic acid produced by lactobacilli may have anti-inflammatory properties (Hearps *et al*., 2017), suggesting that immune modulation by lactobacilli is likely to be multifactorial.

Lactobacillus species are thought to improve vaginal health by promoting epithelial impermeability to pathogens and barrier function in a strain specific manner (Valeriano *et al*., 2014) and producing protective metabolites such as lactic acid and bacteriocins (Aldunate *et al*., 2013; Drissi *et al*, 2015; Hearps *et al*., 2017; Tyssen *et al*., 2018; Pajarillo *et al*., 2015). To maximize the health benefits, *Lactobacillus* strains need be able to adhere to the genital tract epithelium for interaction with host epithelial and immune cells (Jensen *et al*., 2014; Tuo *et al*., 2013). Therefore, the ability of the lactobacilli to adhere to epithelial cells is a critical distinguishing characteristic for selection of strains for probiotics as it provides a distinct advantage for successful colonisation (Buck *et al*., 2005; Montoro *et al*., 2018). Adhesion of lactobacilli to epithelial cells has been described as a complex interaction between surface proteins of lactobacilli and epithelial cells thought to be facilitated by pili on the surface of bacteria (Danne & Dramsi, 2012). It has been shown that removal of lactobacilli surface proteins by treatment with trypsin decreased the adhesive ability of the lactobacilli, highlighting the importance of surface proteins in the adherence of lactobacilli to the host cells (Deepika & Charalampopoulos, 2010; Glenting *et al*., 2013; Zhang *et al*., 2013)

Moreover, Wang *et al.* showed that the addition of surface protein extracts improved the adhesion of strains that initially had poor adhesion ability, highlighting the importance of surface proteins in lactobacilli adhesion (Wang *et al.*, 2018). Additionally, Valeriano *et al.* reported a correlation between lactobacilli adhesion and inhibition of *E. coli in vitro* by pathogen exclusion (Valeriano *et al.*, 2014). To date, proteomic profiling studies have been used to identify several proteins associated with lactobacilli adhesion to epithelial cells (Buck *et al.*, 2005; Jensen *et al.*, 2014; Lorca *et al.*, 2002; Pérez Montoro *et al.*, 2018; Wang *et al.*, 2018; Zhang *et al.*, 2013), including several cell surface components such as polysaccharides and lipoteichoic acids (Deepika & Charalampopoulos, 2010; Yadav *et al.*, 2017). Other adhesins, including collagen-binding protein, mucin-binding protein, surface layer proteins and fibronectin-binding proteins, have also been shown to adhere to extracellular matrix proteins such as collagen, laminin, and fibronectin (Buck *et al.*, 2005; Miyoshi *et al*, 2006; Dhanani & Bagchi, 2013; Deepika & Charalampopoulos, 2010; Wang *et al.*, 2018).

Lactobacilli are constantly exposed to physical and chemical stresses, which induce structural changes in transport proteins, enzymes, and other metabolic changes that may modify the characteristics of the bacteria (reviewed by De Angelis *et al.*, 2016). Analysis of whole-cell protein profiles may be useful for identifying these changes and has also been successfully used in the past to classify microorganisms (Pot *et al*, 1993; Tachedjian *et al.*, 2017; Torriani *et al.*, 1996; Dykes & von Holy, 1994). It is also possible to identify different cell wall protein profiles showing strain-specific patterns even among strains belonging to the same species (Gatti *et al.*, 1997). Here, in order to evaluate differences between lactobacilli isolates that induced low (termed "non-inflammatory") versus high (termed "inflammatory") levels of inflammatory cytokine production, the proteomic profiles of 22 inflammatory and 22 non-inflammatory *Lactobacillus* isolates were analysed using liquid chromatography tandem mass spectrometry (LC-MS/MS) to investigate the underlying mechanisms leading to the different inflammatory profiles.

7.3 Methods

The detailed methodology for proteomic analysis of the vaginal *Lactobacillus* isolates is described in Chapter 2. Sixty-four *Lactobacillus* isolates that were characterised in Chapter 6 were ranked according to the level of inflammatory cytokine production by VK2 cells in response to each isolate. This was determined by combining all proinflammatory cytokines and chemokines assessed onto one component using principal component analysis (PCA) in STATA and generating component estimates for all isolates. Thereafter, the 22 isolates with the highest scores and 22 isolates with the lowest scores were selected to investigate differential protein abundance between the two groups. Briefly, *Lactobacillus* isolates were each cultured in 1.5ml of MRS broth and incubated anaerobically at 37°C for 24 hours. After the incubation, each sample was standardized to $1x10^{12}$ CFU/ml in MRS broth as described in Chapter 2, Section 2.7. The bacterial pellets were each washed 3 times by adding 1ml of sterile PBS into each Eppendorf tube and centrifuging at 10 000rpm for 10 minutes before discarding the supernatant. The supernatant was removed, bacterial pellets were randomized, cells lysed, proteins digested and analyzed using LC-MS/MS analysis at the *Centre for Proteomic and Genomic Research* (CPGR) in Cape Town. Proteins were identified using MaxQuant version 1.5.7.4 against a database including the *Lactobacillus* genus and common contaminants. Protein relative abundance was estimated using intensity-based absolute quantification (iBAQ). Protein functions were determined using aggregated gene ontologies (GO) from UniProt and taxonomy was assigned using UniProt. Protein functions were compared between lactobacilli inducing low inflammation and lactobacilli inducing high inflammation in VK2 cells.

7.4 Results

7.4.1 Description of *Lactobacillus* isolates

The vaginal *Lactobacillus* isolates analysed in this Chapter were obtained from 20 women aged between 16-22 years who participated in the WISH study in Cape Town (Barnabas et al., 2018). The isolates were identified by MALDI-TOF as *L. crispatus* (n=7), *L. jensenii* (n=13), *L. johnsonii* (n=5), *L. mucosae* (n=9), *L. plantarum* (n=1), *L. ruminis* (n=4), *L. salivarius* (n=2) and *L. vaginalis* (n=3). Twenty-six of the lactobacilli isolates analysed in this Chapter were obtained from women who had optimal microbiota (Nugent score 0-3), seven of the isolates were from women with intermediate microbiota (Nugent 4-6), while eleven of the isolates were obtained from women with non-optimal microbiota (Nugent 7-10). All of the women in this sub-study were using hormonal contraceptives at the time of sample collection. Four women were PCR positive for *C. trachomatis* while only two were positive for *N. gonorrhoeae*. All of the women were PCR negative for HSV-1 and 2, *M. genitalium* and *T. pallidum*. The criteria used to select lactobacilli isolates for analysis in this Chapter is shown in **Figure 7.1**. The group that induced low levels of cytokine production included 10 *L. jensenii*, 5 *L. johnsonii*, 4 *L. mucosae*, 1 *L. ruminis*, 2 *L. vaginalis* while isolates that induced high levels of cytokines included 7 *L. crispatus, 3 L. jensenii*, 5 *L. mucosae*, 3 *L. ruminis*, 1 *L. plantarum*, 2 *L. salivarius* and 1 *L. vaginalis.*

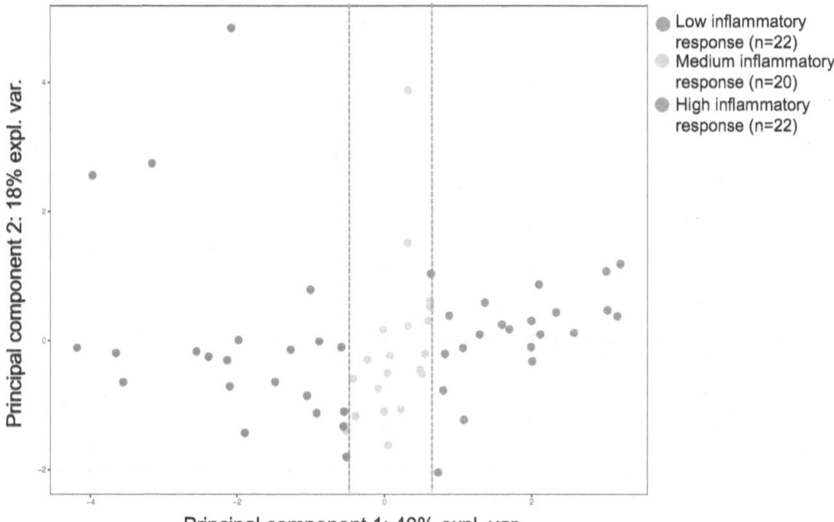

Figure 7.1: Classification of vaginal *Lactobacillus* isolates according to induction of inflammatory cytokine production by VK2 cells. VK2 cell monolayers were cultured to 80% confluency and then treated with *Lactobacillus* isolates (n=64) adjusted to 4.18×10^6 colony forming units (CFU)/ml before being incubated for 24 hours at 37°C with 5% CO_2. Cytokine concentrations in the cell culture supernatants were measured using Luminex. The lactobacilli isolates were ranked according to overall inflammatory cytokine production by the VK2 cells in response to each isolate that was determined by combining all proinflammatory cytokines and chemokines assessed onto one factor using principal component analysis (PCA) in STATA to generate a component estimate for each isolate. The symbols represent lactobacilli isolates.

7.4.2 Assessment of proteomics data quality

Using LC-MS/MS, a total of 5087 *Lactobacillus* proteins were identified from the *Lactobacillus* cultures collectively. Samples were analysed on the MS in multiple batches and these were each processed on different dates. Since processing date has been shown to have on effect on gene expression (Nygaard *et al.*, 2016), variation in protein intensity between batches was evaluated. Inter-batch variation was present between batches processed on different dates and reached significance between the second and fourth batch (**Figure 7.2**). As batch number may have influenced the findings, logistic regression analysis was used to adjust for batch variation in downstream analyses.

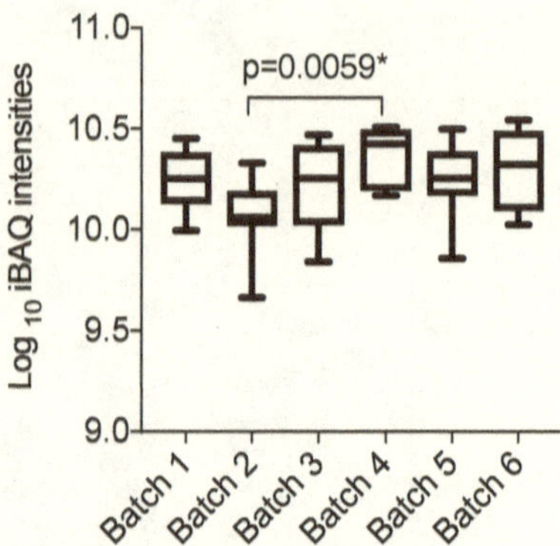

Figure 7.2: Variation in total protein intensities between batches of isolates analysed on different dates on the mass spectrometer. Data are shown as Tukey box plots showing $\log_{10}$-transformed intensity-based absolute quantification (iBAQ) values including [Batch 1 (n=9), Batch 2 (n=7), Batch 3 (n=6), Batch 4 (n=8), Batch 5 (n=8) and Batch 6 (n=6)]. Total iBAQ intensities were determined by the sum of the intensities of all identified proteins per isolate. Boxes represent the interquartile ranges, lines within boxes represent medians and whiskers represent minimum and maximum log-transformed iBAQ intensity values. Mann Whitney U tests were used to compare intensities between batches and p-values were adjusted for multiple comparisons using a false discovery rate step down procedure. *Adjusted p-values <0.05 were considered to be statistically significant.

When the species annotations of the proteins of each strain were evaluated, it was found that all of the isolates expressed *Lactobacillus* proteins that were assigned to more than one *Lactobacillus* species, although in most cases the majority of the proteins were assigned to the correct species (**Figure 7.3 A, B**). This is not surprising due to similarities between *Lactobacillus* proteins between species and database limitations, as a large number of identified proteins were unreviewed, however this finding does highlight the limitations of proteomics for taxonomic assignment.

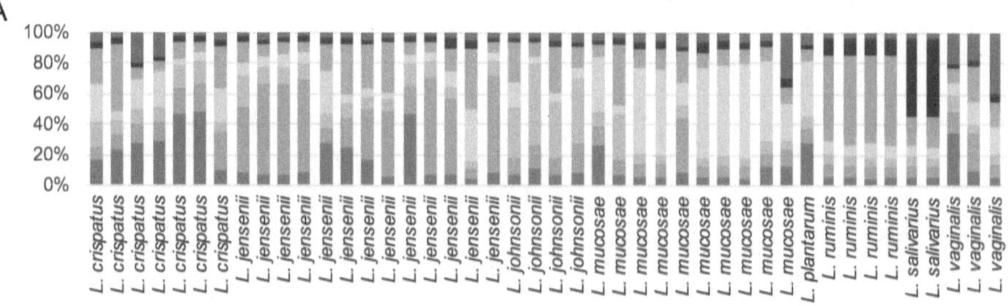

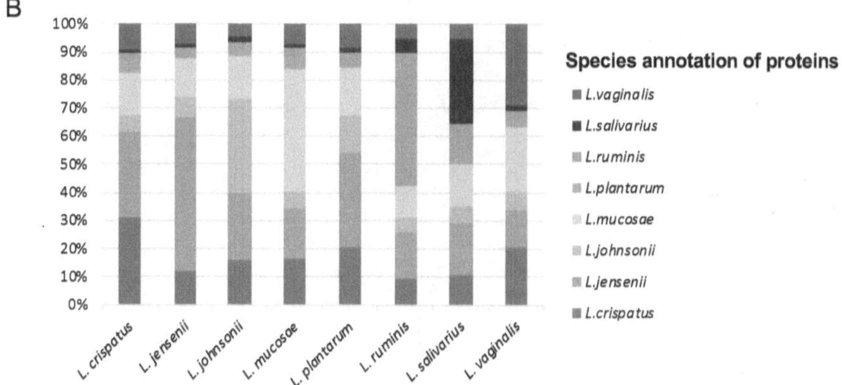

Figure 7.3: Species annotation of lactobacilli proteins detected by mass spectrometry. Vaginal lactobacilli (n=44) were cultured in de Man Rogosa and Sharpe (MRS) broth and incubated at 37°C for 24 hours before being standardised to $1x10^{12}$ CFU/ml in MRS broth. The cultures were centrifuged at high speed for 10min before the supernatant was discarded. Bacterial pellets were washed three times in sterile PBS before protein digestion and liquid chromatography tandem mass spectrometry (LC-MS/MS) analysis. (**A**) Species annotation of proteins identified from individual lactobacilli and (**B**) lactobacilli isolates including [*L. crispatus* (n=7), *L. jensenii* (n=13), *L. johnsonii* (n=4), *L. mucosae* (n=10), *L. plantarum* (n=1), *L. ruminis* (n=4), *L. salivarius* (n=2), and *L. vaginalis* (n=3)] grouped according to species determined using MALDI-TOF Biotyping. The x-axes show the species determined by MALDI-TOF, while the legends show the species annotation of proteins identified using LC-MS/MS.

The overall protein expression patterns of different lactobacilli species were also evaluated using PCA to investigate relationships between species. The analysis showed that proteome profiles differed between lactobacilli species (**Figure 7.4**). There was however a large degree of overlap for *L. crispatus*, *L. jensenii*, *L. johnsonii*, *L. mucosae*, *L. plantarum* and *L. vaginalis* isolates, while

L. ruminis and *L. salivarius* had the most distinct proteome profiles and clustered separately from other species.

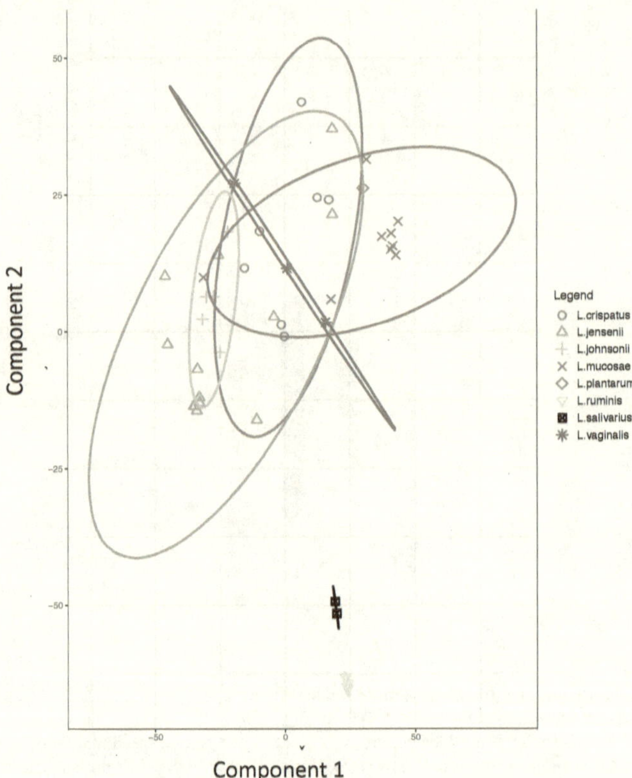

Figure 7.4: Principal component analysis (PCA) showing overall protein expression profiles of eight vaginal *Lactobacillus* species. Vaginal lactobacilli (n=44) including [*L. crispatus* (n=7), *L. jensenii* (n=13), *L. johnsonii* (n=4), *L. mucosae* (n=10), *L. plantarum* (n=1), *L. ruminis* (n=4), *L. salivarius* (n=2), and *L. vaginalis* (n=3)] were cultured in de Man Rogosa and Sharpe (MRS) broth and incubated at 37°C for 24 hours before being standardised to $1x10^{12}$ colony forming units (CFU)/ml in MRS broth. The cultures were centrifuged at high speed for 10min before the supernatant was discarded. Bacterial pellets were washed three times in sterile PBS before protein digestion and liquid chromatography tandem mass spectrometry (LC-MS/MS) analysis. PCA was conducted using the mixOmics package in R. Ellipses represent *Lactobacillus* species.

7.4.3 Identification of differentially abundant proteins between lactobacilli inducing low versus high levels of inflammatory cytokine production by VK2 cells

Total iBAQ intensities and intensities of individual proteins were compared between *Lactobacillus* isolates that induced high versus low inflammatory responses in VK2 cells. Interestingly, it was found that, even though the same amount of total protein was processed for LC-MS/MS analysis for each sample, lactobacilli that induced low levels of inflammatory cytokine responses had a significantly higher protein relative abundance compared to less inflammatory isolates (**Figure 7.5**). Overall protein expression was compared between high and low inflammatory cytokine-inducing isolates using PCA. Proteins grouped on Component 1 explained 16% of the overall variance, while those grouped on Component 2 explained 15% of the variance (**Figure 7.6**). Although there was a large degree of similarity and hence overlap between the groups, clustering of the isolates that induced less inflammatory cytokine production higher on Component 1 suggests over-representation of proteins associated with Component 1 in less inflammatory isolates (**Figure 7.6**).

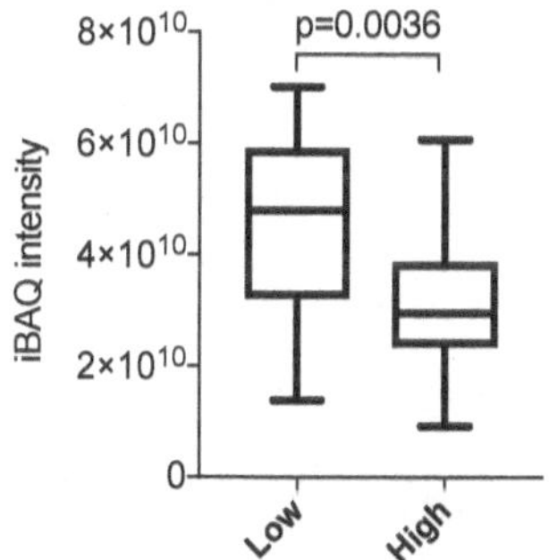

Figure 7.5: Comparison of protein iBAQ intensities between vaginal lactobacilli inducing low levels of inflammatory cytokine production (n=22) and isolates inducing high levels of inflammatory cytokine (n=22) production in VK2 cells. Vaginal lactobacilli (n=44) were cultured in de Man Rogosa and Sharpe (MRS) broth and incubated at 37°C for 24 hours before being standardised to 1×10^{12} CFU/ml in MRS broth. The cultures were centrifuged at high speed for 10min before the supernatant was discarded. Bacterial pellets were washed three times in sterile PBS before protein digestion and liquid chromatography tandem mass spectrometry (LC-MS/MS) analysis. Data are shown as Tukey box plots showing $\log_{10}$-transformed intensity-based absolute quantification (iBAQ) values. Total iBAQ intensities were determined by the sum of all identified protein intensities per isolate. Boxes represent the interquartile ranges, lines within boxes represent medians and whiskers represent minimum and maximum $\log_{10}$-transformed iBAQ intensity values. Mann Whitney U test was used to compare intensities and a p-value <0.05 was considered to be statistically significant.

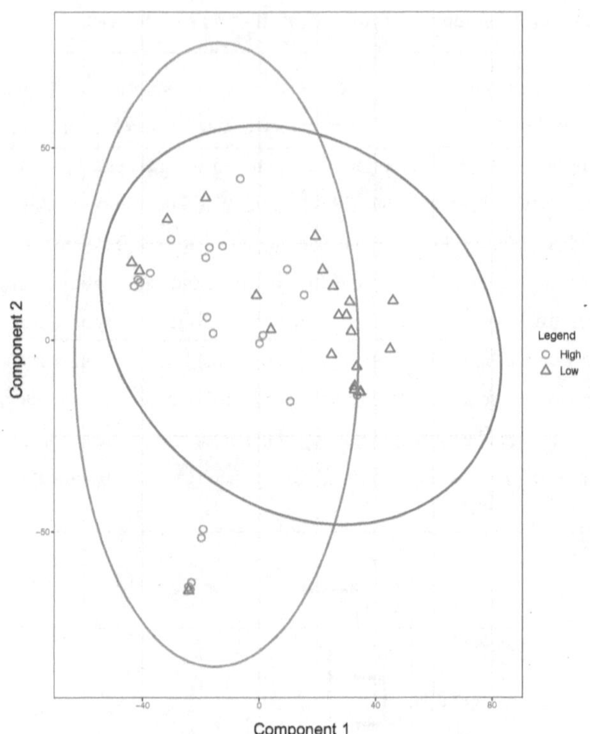

Figure 7.6: Principal component analysis of proteins extracted from vaginal lactobacilli isolates inducing low (n=22) and high (n=22) levels of inflammatory cytokine production by VK2 cells. Vaginal lactobacilli (n=44) were cultured in de Man Rogosa and Sharpe (MRS) broth and incubated at 37°C for 24 hours before being standardised to $1x10^{12}$ CFU/ml in MRS broth. The cultures were centrifuged at high speed for 10 min before the supernatant was discarded. Bacterial pellets were washed three times in sterile phosphate buffered saline (PBS) before protein digestion and liquid chromatography tandem mass spectrometry (LC-MS/MS) analysis. Proteins were identified in MaxQuant by searching mass spectra against a sub-database of Uniprot including proteins from the *Lactobacillus* genus and common contaminants. Each point represents an individual *Lactobacillus* isolate. The distribution of the isolates is based on proteins and the distance between samples represents similarity between the proteomes of the isolates. Principal component analysis (PCA) was conducted using the mixOmics package in R.

Using the limma R package, it was found that a total of 164 proteins were differentially abundant between lactobacilli inducing low inflammatory cytokine production and those inducing high levels of inflammatory cytokines in VK2 cells (**Figure 7.7 and Appendix IV**).

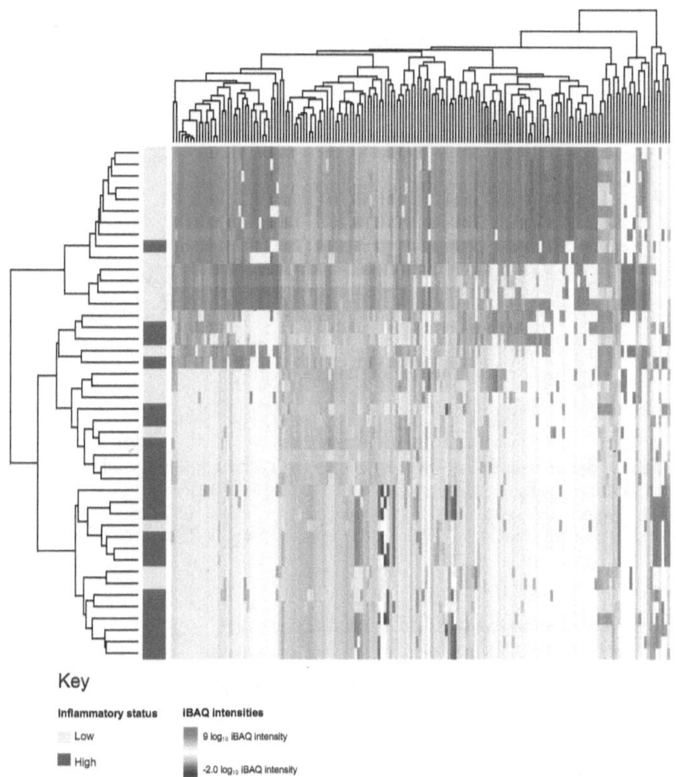

Figure 7.7: Heatmap of differentially abundant proteins between vaginal *Lactobacillus* isolates that induced high (n=22) versus low (n=22) inflammatory responses. Vaginal lactobacilli (n=44) were cultured in de Man Rogosa and Sharpe (MRS) broth and incubated at 37°C for 24 hours before being standardised to $1x10^{12}$ CFU/ml in MRS broth. The cultures were centrifuged at high speed for 10min before the supernatant was discarded. Bacterial pellets were washed three times in sterile phosphate buffered saline (PBS) before protein digestion and liquid chromatography tandem mass spectrometry (LC-MS/MS) analysis. Proteins were identified in MaxQuant by searching mass spectra against a sub-database of Uniprot including proteins from the *Lactobacillus* genus and common contaminants. Differentially abundant proteins between lactobacilli inducing low vs high inflammatory cytokine responses in VK2 cells were identified using the limma R package.

The majority of the proteins were under-represented (157/164) in isolates that induced high inflammatory responses compared to those that induced low levels of cytokine production in VK2 cells. Most of these proteins were assigned to *L. jensenii* and *L. johnsonii* species (**Figure 7.8**), which is not surprising given that the group of isolates that induced low levels of inflammatory cytokine production included a greater number of these species.

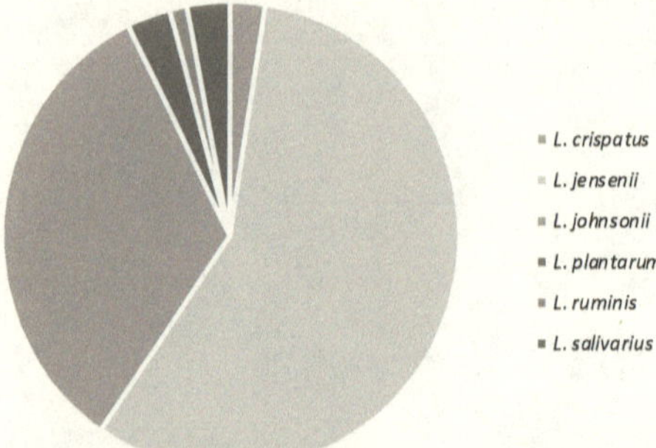

Figure 7.8: Pie chart showing the distribution of species annotation of differentially abundant lactobacilli proteins. The majority of the differentially abundant proteins were assigned to *L. jensenii* (n=93) and *L. johnsonii* (n=54), while the rest were assigned to *L. crispatus* (n=4), *L. plantarum* (n=5), *L. ruminis* (n=3) and *L. salivarius* (n=5). Differentially abundant proteins were identified using the limma package in R.

7.4.4 *Lactobacillus* functions associated with inflammatory profiles

As the distribution of species was uneven between the high and low inflammation groups, further analysis was conducted using GO functional annotation. Each protein was assigned to a biological process, a cellular localization and a molecular function, based on information from the GO database and GO annotations were then aggregated.

The biological processes that were over-represented in isolates inducing high inflammatory responses included those involved with *de novo* inosine monophosphate (IMP) biosynthetic process (0.47-log fold change) and protein complex oligomerization (0.47-log fold change; **Table 7.1**). The majority of the under-represented GO categories were involved with biosynthetic processes, metabolic processes, and transportation (**Figure 7.9A**) and these included teichoic acid biosynthetic process (-0.43-log fold change), cobalamin biosynthetic process (-0.30-log fold change), riboflavin biosynthetic process (-0.27-log fold change), peptide metabolic process (-0.47-log fold change), coenzyme A metabolic process (-0.46-log fold change), nucleotide metabolic process (-0.44-log fold change), nucleoside metabolic process (-0.42-log fold change), intracellular protein transmembrane transport (-0.37-log fold change), transmembrane transport (-0.22-log fold change) and peptide transport (-0.19-log fold change; **Table 7.1).**

All the cellular components were under-represented in lactobacilli inducing high inflammatory cytokine responses (**Table 7.2**) and included (i) extrinsic component of plasma membrane (-1.67-log fold change); (ii) bacterial nucleoid (-0.98-log fold change); ATP binding cassette transporter complex (-0.21-log fold change); plasma membrane (-0.14-log fold change), integral component of membrane (-0.16-log fold change) and chromosome (-0.13-log fold change; **Table 7.2**). Of the six cellular components that were associated with inflammatory profile, half (3/6) were membrane components (**Figure 7.9B**).

Arginine binding was the only molecular function that was over-represented in lactobacilli inducing high inflammation, while the majority were under-represented 23/24 (**Table 7.3**). A total of 16/24 molecular functions that were differentially expressed between isolates that induced low versus high inflammatory responses were involved in enzymatic activity including metallopeptidase, endoribonuclease, exonuclease, arginine-tRNA ligase, adenine deaminase, carbamoyl-phosphate synthase, hydrolase activity, hydroxymethylglutaryl-CoA synthase, methylthioadenosine nucleosidase and transferases. A total of 5/24 of the differentially abundant molecular functions were classified as being involved with binding activity, including calcium ion binding, coenzyme binding, transition metal ion binding, DNA-binding transcription factor activity and carbohydrate derivative binding (**Figure 7.9C**). The remainder of the molecular functions were involved in transporter activity (**Figure 7.9C**).

A

protein flavinylation 4%
protein import 4%
rRNA base methylation 4%
phosphoenolpyruvatedependent sugar phosphotransferase system 4%
protein complex oligomerization 4%
biosynthetic processes 17%
protein targeting 4%
chromosome segregation 4%
metabolic processes 17%
catabolic processes 4%
DNA repair and transcription 14%
transportation 14%
translation 8%

B

bacterial nucleoid 17%
extrinsic component of plasma membrane 16%
ATP-binding cassette (ABC) transporter complex 17%
integral component of membrane 16%
chromosome 17%
plasma membrane 17%

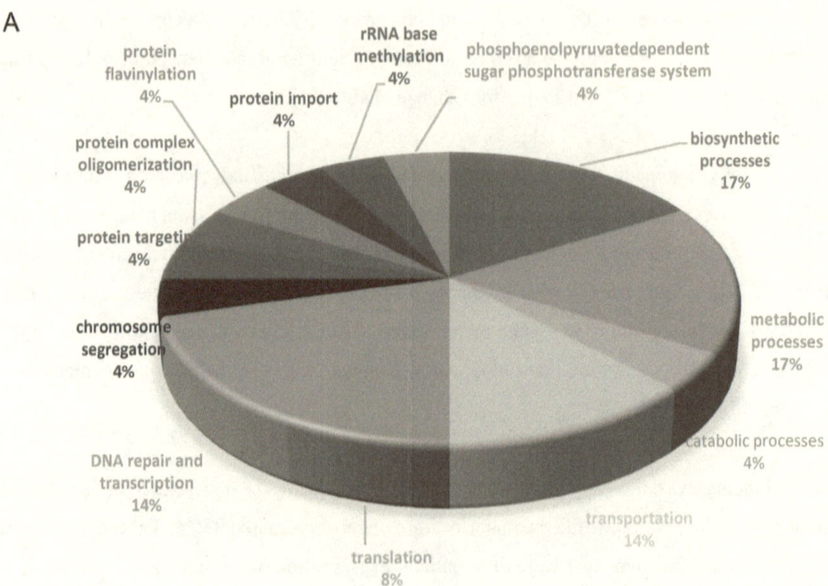

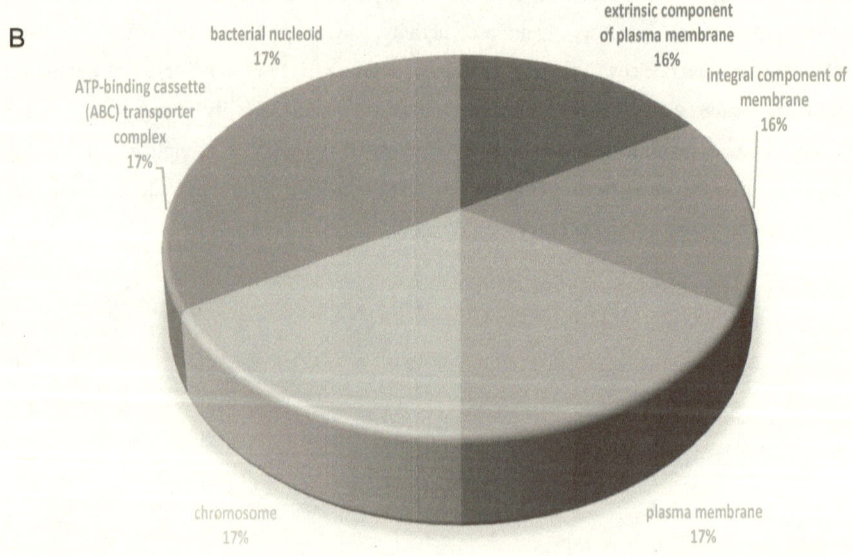

C

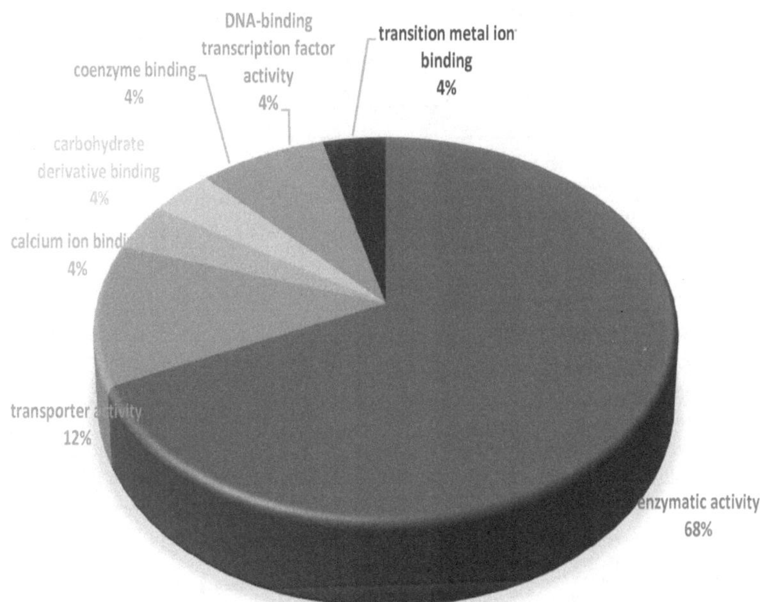

Figure 7.9: Pie charts illustrating the gene ontology (GO) categories that were differentially abundant between vaginal lactobacilli inducing low (n=22) versus high (n=22) inflammatory responses in VK2 cells. Differentially abundant (A) biological processes (B) cellular components and (C) molecular functions are shown. GOs for each protein were determined using Uniprot and the intensity-based absolute quantification (iBAQ) values for all proteins with a particular GO were then aggregated. The R limma package was used to determine differentially abundant GOs between isolates inducing low versus high inflammatory responses.

The molecular functions that demonstrated the greatest under-representation included calcium transmembrane transporter activity (-1.79-log fold change), ATPase-coupled organic phosphonate transmembrane transporter activity (-1.68-log fold change), deoxyribonuclease activity (-1.38-log fold change), rRNA (cytosine-N-4-)-methyltransferase activity, endonuclease activity (-1.34-log fold change), DNA N-glycosylase activity (-1.34-log fold change) and glycerol-3-phopshate cytidylyltransferase activity (-1.34-log fold change).

Table 7.1. Differentially abundant biological processes between inflammatory and non-inflammatory vaginal *Lactobacillus* isolates

Biological process	logFC	AveExpr	t	P.Value	adj.P.Val	B
Peptide metabolic process	-0.47	0.48	-4.00	0.00022398	0.03179913	0.51
rRNA base methylation	-0.47	0.62	-4.15	0.00013816	0.03179913	0.96
DNA restriction modification system	-0.46	0.53	-3.45	0.00119865	0.03870969	-1.01
Coenzyme A metabolic process	-0.46	0.71	-3.51	0.00100213	0.03870969	-0.85
Purine nucleoside triphosphate catabolic process	-0.44	0.68	-3.40	0.00136945	0.03870969	-1.13
Nucleotide metabolic process	-0.44	0.68	-3.40	0.00136945	0.03870969	-1.13
Teichoic acid biosynthetic process	-0.43	0.52	-3.73	0.00052499	0.03179913	-0.26
Nucleoside metabolic process	-0.42	0.77	-3.31	0.00178034	0.04213727	-1.36
Protein flavinylation	-0.40	0.39	-3.61	0.00073397	0.03870969	-0.57
Protein import	-0.37	1.06	-3.51	0.00101193	0.03870969	-0.86
Protein targeting	-0.37	1.18	-3.25	0.00215852	0.04213727	-1.54
Intracellular protein transmembrane transport	-0.37	1.18	-3.25	0.00215852	0.04213727	-1.54
Trans-translation	-0.36	0.56	-3.77	0.00045153	0.03179913	-0.12
Chromosome segregation	-0.35	0.81	-3.15	0.00283922	0.04815321	-1.78
Negative regulation of transcription DNA templated	-0.32	0.96	-3.75	0.0004903	0.03179913	-0.20
Cobalamin biosynthetic process	-0.30	0.64	-3.29	0.00191125	0.04213727	-1.43
Riboflavin biosynthetic process	-0.27	0.16	-3.24	0.00218637	0.04213727	-1.55
Transmembrane transport	-0.22	1.84	-3.93	0.00027661	0.03179913	0.32
Peptide transport	-0.19	1.32	-3.31	0.00182587	0.04213727	-1.39
DNA repair	-0.18	1.33	-3.21	0.00242608	0.04472428	-1.64
Positive regulation of translation	-0.17	0.88	-3.18	0.00260099	0.04595079	-1.70
Phosphoenolpyruvate dependent sugar phosphotransferase system	-0.16	2.05	-3.46	0.00115064	0.03870969	-0.97
de novo IMP biosynthetic process	0.47	0.96	3.36	0.00156418	0.04145068	-1.25
Protein complex oligomerization	0.47	0.52	3.51	0.0010025	0.03870969	-0.85

logFC, log fold change; AveExpr, average log2 expression; t, t-statistic; P.value, raw p-value; adj.P.val, adjusted p-value; B, log odds that the gene is differentially expressed

Table 7.2. Differentially abundant cellular components between inflammatory and non-inflammatory vaginal *Lactobacillus* isolates

Cellular components	logFC	AveExpr	t	P.Value	adj.P.Val	B
Extrinsic component of plasma membrane	-1.67	-0.67	-4.92	1.32E-05	0.0008312	3.01
Bacterial nucleoid	-0.98	0.31	-3.01	0.00434186	0.03907677	-2.45
ATP binding cassette (ABC) transporter complex	-0.21	1.78	-3.05	0.00388753	0.03907677	-2.35
Integral component of membrane	-0.17	2.66	-4.42	6.49E-05	0.00204342	1.49
Plasma membrane	-0.15	2.21	-3.99	0.00025271	0.00530688	0.20
Chromosome	-0.13	1.71	-3.52	0.00102127	0.01608498	-1.11

logFC, log fold change; AveExpr, average log2 expression; t, t-statistic; P.value, raw p-value; adj.P.val, adjusted p-value; B, log odds that the gene is differentially expressed

Table 7.3. Differentially abundant molecular functions between inflammatory and non-inflammatory vaginal *Lactobacillus* isolates

Molecular function	logFC	AveExpr	t	P.Value	adj.P.Val	B
Calcium transmembrane transporter activity, phosphorylative mechanism	-1.79	-0.24	-5.97	3.91E-07	0.00028395	6.36
ATPase-coupled organic phosphonate transmembrane transporter activity	-1.68	-0.66	-4.92	1.30E-05	0.00472593	3.14
Type I site-specific deoxyribonuclease activity	-1.48	-1.01	-4.55	4.28E-05	0.00777312	2.04
rRNA (cytosine-N-4-)-methyltransferase activity	-1.38	-0.01	-3.85	0.00038637	0.03779056	0.03
Class I DNA-(apurinic or apyrimidinic site) endonuclease activity	-1.34	-0.95	-3.62	0.00077435	0.03779056	-0.60
DNA N-glycosylase activity	-1.34	-0.95	-3.62	0.00077435	0.03779056	-0.60
Glycerol-3-phosphate cytidylyltransferase activity	-1.34	-0.30	-3.53	0.00098333	0.03779056	-0.81
Hydroxymethylglutaryl-CoA reductase activity	-1.29	-0.22	-3.58	0.00086988	0.03779056	-0.70
Branched-chain amino acid transmembrane transporter activity	-1.28	-1.24	-3.93	0.00030307	0.03672241	0.25
N-acetyl glucosaminyl diphosphoundecaprenol N-acetyl-beta-D-mannosaminyltransferase activity	-1.26	-0.62	-3.40	0.00144317	0.04503991	-1.16
Acylphosphatase activity	-1.26	0.03	-3.56	0.00091277	0.03779056	-0.74
Methylenetetrahydrofolatet RNA uracil-5-methyltransferase FADH2 oxidizing activity	-1.24	-0.12	-3.39	0.00148687	0.04503991	-1.18
5',10-methylenetetrahydrofolatedependent tRNA (m5U54) methyltransferase activity	-1.24	-0.12	-3.39	0.00148687	0.04503991	-1.18
ATPase-coupled transmembrane transporter activity	-1.14	0.58	-3.78	0.00047214	0.03779056	-0.15
Transferase activity transferring glycosyl groups	-1.10	0.14	-3.53	0.00099354	0.03779056	-0.82
Ornithine decarboxylase activity	-0.99	0.40	-3.52	0.001031	0.03779056	-0.85
Endonuclease activity	-0.30	1.22	-3.35	0.00165826	0.04822207	-1.28
Catalytic activity	-0.27	1.64	-4.61	3.50E-05	0.00777312	2.23
Metalloendopeptidase activity	-0.26	1.31	-3.66	0.00068613	0.03779056	-0.49
Carbohydrate binding	-0.24	1.54	-3.97	0.00026701	0.03672241	0.37
Hydrolase activity	-0.19	2.14	-3.63	0.00073891	0.03779056	-0.55
Transferase activity	-0.16	1.65	-3.56	0.00090315	0.03779056	-0.74
ATPase activity	-0.16	2.38	-3.50	0.00109161	0.03779056	-0.91
Arginine binding	1.47	-0.44	3.70	0.00060623	0.03779056	-0.37

logFC, log fold change; AveExpr, average log2 expression; t, t-statistic; P.value, raw p-value; adj.P.val, adjusted p-value; B, log odds that the gene is differentially expressed

Logistic regression was also carried out to evaluate the relationships observed between GOs and inflammatory responses to the *Lactobacillus* isolates, adjusting for possible confounders including batch number and species. Functional categories and the adjusted p-values are shown in **Table 7.4**. It was found that all associations between the inflammatory nature of the *Lactobacillus* isolates and cellular components while 21/24 molecular functions and 15/24 biological processes remained significant after adjusting for batch number and species.

Table 7.4. Logistic regression analysis of relationships between gene ontologies and inflammatory cytokine responses

Gene ontology	β-coefficient	95% confidence interval	p-value
Cellular components			
Extrinsic component of plasma	-1.04	-1.60 - -0.48	<0.001
Integral component of membrane	-7.82	-13.21- -2.44	0.004
Plasma membrane	-10.83	-17.66 - -4.00	0.002
ATP-binding cassette (ABC) transporter complex	-5.49	-9.71- -1.28	0.011
Bacterial nucleoid	-1.79	-3.07 - -0.50	0.006
Molecular functions			
Calcium transmembrane transporter activity, phosphorylative mechanism	-1.80	-2.87 - -0.74	0.001
ATPase-coupled organic phosphonate transmembrane transporter activity	-1.03	-1.59 - -0.47	<0.001
Catalytic activity	-4.72	-9.13 - -0.30	0.036
Type I site-specific deoxyribonuclease activity	-1.12	-1.79 - -0.46	0.001
Branched-chain amino acid transmembrane transporter activity	-1.10	-1.90 - -0.312	0.006
rRNA (cytosine-N4-)-methyltransferase activity	-1.06	-1.75 - -0.36	0.003
Arginine binding	0.92	0.33 -1.51	0.002
ATPase-coupled transmembrane transporter activity	-3.72	-6.86- -0.58	0.020
Metallopeptidase activity	-3.68	-7.69 - 0.34	0.073
Class I DNA-(apurinic or apyrimidinic site) endonuclease activity	-0.83	-1.38 - -0.28	0.003
DNA N-glycosylase activity	-0.83	-1.38 - -0.28	0.003
5'10'-methylenetetrahydrofolate-dependent tRNA (m5U54) methyltransferase activity	-0.76	-1.30 - -0.23	0.005
Hydroxymethylglutaryl-CoA synthase activity	-0.54	-1.10 - 0.03	0.063
Transferase activity	-14.25	-23.27 - -5.22	0.002
Acylphosphatase activity	-1.29	-2.18 - -0.41	0.004
Glycerol-3-phosphate cytidylyltransferase activity	-1.17	-1.99 - -0.36	0.005
Transferase activity, transferring glycosyl groups	-0.66	-1.27 - -0.05	0.034
Ornithine decarboxylase activity	-7.38	-13.97 - -0.79	0.028
Metalloendopeptidase activity	-6.32	-10.63 - -2.01	0.004
ATPase activity	-10.66	-17.55 - -3.77	0.002
N-acetylglucosaminyldiphosphoundecaprenol N-acetyl-beta-D-mannosaminyltransferase activity	-0.82	-1.37 - -0.26	0.004
Methylenetetrahydrofolate-tRNA-(uracil-5-)-methyltransferase (FADH2-oxidizing) activity	-0.76	-1.30 - -0.23	0.005
Endonuclease activity	-3.50	-5.92 - -1.08	0.005
Hydrolase activity	-1.40	-4.64 - 1.90	0.411
Carbohydrate binding	0.24	-0.26 - 0.74	0.344

Biological process	β-coefficient	95% confidence interval	p-value
Chromosome segregation	-3.00	-5.25 - -0.75	0.009
Coenzyme A metabolic process	-3.26	-5.48 -1.03	0.004
DNA restriction modification system	-2.06	-3.45 - -0.66	0.004
Intracellular protein transmembrane transport	-4.07	-7.66 - -0.48	0.026
Negative regulation of transcription-DNA templated	-7.36	-12.24- -2.48	0.003
Nucleotide metabolic process	-2.64	-5.15 - -0.13	0.039
Peptide metabolic process	-2.70	-4.37 - -1.02	0.002
Positive regulation of translation	-5.72	-9.64 - -1.80	0.004
Protein complex oligomerization	2.46	0.82 - 4.09	0.003
Protein flavinylation	-3.35	-5.53 - -1.18	0.003
Protein import	-4.21	-7.49 - -0.92	0.012
Protein target	-4.07	-7.66- -0.48	0.026
Purine nucleoside triphosphate catabolic process	-2.82	-4.77 - -0.87	0.005
rRNA base methylation	-3.50	-5.70 - -1.30	0.002
Trans-translation	-3.62	-6.07 - 1.18	0.004
Glutathione transmembrane transport	0.81	-1.41 - 3.03	0.474
Teichoic acid biosynthetic process	0.22	-1.09 - 1.53	0.742
Riboflavin biosynthetic process	-0.66	-2.30 - 0.98	0.429
Phosphoenolpyruvate-dependent phosphotransferase system	-1.72	-3.89 -0.45	0.121
Oligopeptide transport	2.70	-0.26 - 5.67	0.074
Nucleoside metabolic process	2.37	-6.17 -1.42	0.220
DNA repair	-2.09	-5.44 - 1.26	0.222
De novo IMP biosynthetic process	-0.30	-1.80 - 1.21	0.700
Cobalamin biosynthetic process	3.07	-0.49 - 6.62	0.091

7.4.5 Relationships between lactobacilli biotherapeutic-relevant characteristics and proteome profiles

Since lactobacilli adhesion to epithelial cells has been associated with the protective nature of the bacteria in the FGT, the relationship between cell adhesion protein expression and the level of lactobacilli adhesion to VK2 cells was investigated. Potential cell adhesion proteins including surface protein aggregation promoting factor, cell surface protein, bacterial surface layer protein fragment, surface anchor protein, cell surface protein ErfK/YbiS/YcfS/YnhG family, cell surface protein CscC family, cell surface protein CscB family, cell surface protein CscB family, cell surface protein lipoprotein, cell surface protein LPXTG-motif cell wall anchor, sortase-anchored surface protein, Rib/alpha/Esp surface antigen, mucin binding protein LPXTG-motif cell wall anchor were identified using LC-MS/MS and the association between the adhesion proteins and lactobacilli adhesion to VK2 cells *in vitro* was determined using Spearman's correlation analysis. Surface protein aggregation promoting factor (Spearman rho=0.3137; p=0.0381) was positively correlated with the level of adhesion to VK2 cells, although the relationship was not upheld after adjusting for batch number and species [β-coefficient: 0.12; 95% confidence interval (CI): -0.44-0.20; p=0.446)].

On the other hand, cell surface protein (Spearman rho=-0.1936; p=0.2080), bacterial surface layer protein fragment (Spearman rho=-0.2063; p=0.1791), surface anchor protein (Spearman rho=0.08086; p=0.6018), cell surface protein ErfK/YbiS/YcfS/YnhG family (Spearman rho=0.1319; p=0.3934), cell surface protein, CscC family (Spearman rho=-0.1459; p=0.3446), cell surface protein, CscB family (Spearman rho=-0.01033; p=0.9469), cell surface protein, lipoprotein (Spearman rho=-0.1823; p=0.2363), cell surface protein LPXTG-motif cell wall anchor (Spearman rho=-0.06803; p=0.6608), sortase-anchored surface protein (Spearman rho=0.1182; p=0.4447), Rib/alpha/Esp surface antigen (Spearman rho=0.2426; p=0.1125) and mucin binding protein LPXTG-motif cell wall anchor (Spearman rho= 0.02784; p= 0.8576) did not correlate significantly with the level of adhesion.

Additionally, since strongly adherent lactobacilli induced production of low levels of inflammatory cytokines in VK2 cells (Chapter 6), proteome profiles were compared between highly adherent and weakly adherent lactobacilli using the limma package in R. It was found that ribonucleoside-triphosphate reductase (β-coefficient: -0.43; 95% confidence interval (CI): -0.66--0.19; p<0.001) and UPF0342 protein LRC_11170 (β-coefficient: -0.35; 95% confidence interval (CI): -0.56--0.15 p=0.001) were differentially abundant after adjusting for batch number and species.

The production of D-lactate by lactobacilli isolates correlated positively with D-lactate dehydrogenase protein relative abundance (Spearman rho=0.3457; p=0.0215), while a trend towards a positive correlation was observed between L-lactate production and L-lactate dehydrogenase relative abundance (Spearman rho=0.2754; p=0.0700). A strong negative correlation was found between D-lactate dehydrogenase relative abundance and inflammatory cytokine response PCA scores (Spearman rho=-0.4567; p=0.0018), while L-lactate dehydrogenase relative abundance were not significantly associated with PCA scores (Spearman rho=-0.1040; p= 0.5016).

7.5 Discussion

Studies have shown that upregulated levels of inflammatory cytokines in the FGT are associated with an increased HIV acquisition risk in women (Morrison *et al.*, 2014; Masson *et al.*, 2015). *Lactobacillus* species may protect against HIV acquisition, other STIs and non-optimal microbiota by producing metabolites such as lactic acid, hydrogen peroxide and bacteriocins and by competing for adhesion sites (Gong *et al.*, 2014; Aldunate *et al.*, 2015; El-Adawi *et al.*, 2015; Gosmann *et al.*, 2017; Hearps *et al.*, 2017; Arena *et al.*, 2018). Additionally, lactobacilli appear to modulate inflammatory responses in the FGT (Anahtar *et al.*, 2015; Gosmann *et al.*, 2017). It has also been shown that the protective characteristics of lactobacilli may differ between different lactobacilli species, as well as between strains within species, but the mechanisms underlying these differences remain unclear. In this Chapter, MS was used to identify lactobacilli protein signatures associated with inflammatory cytokine production by VK2 cells in response to stimulation with *Lactobacillus* isolates, as well as lactobacilli adhesion to VK2 cells. Interestingly, lactobacilli isolates that induced low levels of inflammatory cytokine production had a significantly higher total protein relative abundance compared to isolates that induced high levels of inflammatory responses in VK2 cells, even though the same amount of protein was analyzed for each isolate. When PCA was used to compare overall protein expression, there was a large degree of overlap between isolates that induced high versus low inflammatory responses, likely due to similarities in the majority of proteins between the isolates. Of the 5087 proteins detected, 164 were differentially abundant between lactobacilli inducing low versus high levels of inflammatory cytokine production by VK2 cells, with the majority of the proteins assigned to *L. jensenii* and *L. johnsonii* species. Functional analysis revealed that 3/6 of the cellular components that were underabundant in inflammatory isolates were membrane-associated. The majority of the molecular functions that were underabundant in inflammatory isolates were enzymatic pathways, suggesting that the less inflammatory isolates had greater metabolic activity. The ribonucleoside-triphosphate reductase enzyme and UPF0342 protein LRC_11170 were differentially abundant between lactobacilli that were highly adherent versus less adherent lactobacilli, while surface protein aggregation promotion factor correlated positively with lactobacilli adhesion to VK2 cells. Production of D-lactate was positively correlated with D-lactate dehydrogenase relative abundance, which was strongly inversely associated with inflammatory cytokine responses.

The ability of lactobacilli to survive in different ecological niches may be attributed to the ability of the species to adapt (De Angelis *et al.*, 2016). Previous studies have demonstrated modifications of *Lactobacillus* proteins belonging to various functional categories, including carbohydrate transport and metabolism (Bove *et al.*, 2012; Siragusa *et al.*, 2014), pyruvate metabolism (Koponen *et al.*, 2012; Zhai *et al.*, 2014), proteolytic system, amino acid metabolism, protein synthesis (Laakso *et al.*, 2011; Bove *et al.*, 2012; Al-Naseri *et al.*, 2013; Wang *et al.*, 2013), nucleotide metabolism, lipid transport (Cohen *et al.*, 2006; Laakso *et al.*, 2011; Rivas-Sendra *et al.*, 2011; Al-Naseri *et al.*, 2013), metabolism, cell wall and extracellular proteins as lactobacilli adapt to different environmental niches or stresses. Genomic analysis was also used to demonstrate that bacterial adaptation was associated with the tendency to simplify metabolic processes (Cai *et al.*, 2009; Goh & Klaenhammer, 2009). Here, it was also shown that the majority of the proteins were under-represented in isolates that induced high levels of cytokine responses and were mostly assigned to *L. jensenii* and *L. johnsonii*. Since the distribution of the species was uneven, the GO functional annotations (which were obtained by grouping each protein with a particular function, regardless of species) were also analysed and compared between lactobacilli that induced low versus high inflammatory responses. Molecular functional categories involved with proteolytic systems, nucleotide metabolism, transmembrane transport, transferase activity, oxidative phosphorylation, catalytic activity and carbohydrate metabolism were over-abundant in lactobacilli inducing low versus high inflammatory responses after adjusting for batch number and species. Additionally, biological processes including biosynthetic processes, catabolic processes, translation, chromosome segregation, protein targeting, rRNA base methylation and DNA restriction modification system were also over-abundant in less inflammatory isolates. These findings suggest that less inflammatory isolates may have greater metabolic activity. It has previously been shown that lactobacilli protein expression may be significantly downregulated at pH ranges associated with non-optimal microbiomes (>4.5) (Borgdorff *et al.*, 2016), suggesting that lactobacilli isolated from women with non-optimal microbiota may have reduced metabolic activity. A decline in metabolic activity may result in reduced production of lactic acid, the main lactobacilli metabolite that acidifies the FGT. This may also explain the inflammatory nature of the isolates since lactic acid has been described as one of the most important lactobacilli metabolite that has anti-inflammatory properties (Hearps *et al.*, 2017) and D-lactate, as well as D-lactate dehydrogenase which also were found to be inversely associated with inflammatory cytokine production in the present study. Of note, the pH of the *Lactobacillus* cultures was not associated with inflammatory responses, suggesting that any adaption as a result of pH that may have occurred was not due to *in vitro* conditions. As described in Chapter 6 of this book, lactobacilli isolated from women with non-optimal microbiota were more inflammatory and produced less lactic acid than those isolated from women with optimal microbiota. Taken together, these findings suggest that high pH in women with non-optimal microbiota may result in the adaption of *Lactobacillus* species, including reduced metabolic activity and lactic acid production, that in turn hinders the immunomodulatory abilities of these isolates. Alternatively, the inherent properties of the lactobacilli present in the FGT may influence the potential for non-optimal bacteria to colonize this compartment. These findings suggest that functional proteomics analysis illustrating the modifications that occur in lactobacilli species during environmental changes may be useful for the screening for strains with optimal characteristics for use in probiotic formulations.

Additionally, an overabundance of membrane cellular components in less inflammatory isolates suggests that the majority of the differentially abundant proteins were localised to the membrane. This in turn may indicate that interaction between the *Lactobacillus* membrane and host cells, as well as membrane transport systems, play an important role in modulating inflammatory responses. This was not surprising as it has previously been reported that cell wall proteins, as well as the cell membrane, may influence the immunomodulatory properties of *Lactobacillus* species (Kulakauskas & Marie-Pierre Chapot-Chartier, 2014). Although, most of the differentially abundant molecular functions and biological processes were under-represented in lactobacilli inducing high inflammatory responses, proteins involved with arginine binding, an amino acid that is involved in protein synthesis, was over-represented, suggesting an increase in protein synthesis in isolates inducing high inflammation.

Previous studies have reported differences in lactobacilli properties between species (Osset *et al*., 2001; Sanders, 2008; Verstraelen *et al*., 2009). Additionally, in Chapter 6, a large variation in inflammatory properties was observed between lactobacilli species, as well as between strains of particular species, when lactobacilli isolates were co-cultured with VK2 cells *in vitro*. Here, proteome profiles were also compared between lactobacilli species to evaluate relationships between the species. As expected, it was found that different species had different proteome profiles, although there was a great degree of overlap between *L. crispatus*, *L. jensenii*, *L. johnsonii*, *L. mucosae*, *L. vaginalis* and *L. plantarum*. This may have been due to similarities between conserved, housekeeping *Lactobacillus* proteins between these species. On the other hand, *L. salivarius* and *L. ruminis* species clustered separately from all the other species analysed. This may reflect the fact that these species are less commonly isolated from the FGT compared to the other lactobacilli species and may possess different functional properties (Pavlova *et al.*, 2002; Ravel *et al.*, 2011; Pendharkar *et al.*, 2013; Anahtar *et al.*, 2015; Gosmann *et al.*, 2017; Lennard *et al.*, 2017; Onywera *et al.*, 2019; Pino *et al.*, 2019). Interestingly, a wide distribution of some strains within particular species, for example *L. jensenii* and *L. mucosae*, was observed, suggesting significant diversity among strains within these species. It has been shown that the distribution of proteins involved in amino acid or carbohydrate transport and metabolism varies among *Lactobacillus* species (Goh & Klaenhammer, 2009). Additionally, proteins involved with carbohydrate transport can also vary between strains of the same species as has been shown for *L. plantarum* and *L. rhamnosus* (Bove *et al.*, 2012; Siragusa *et al.*, 2014). However, in this Chapter, relatively small numbers of each strain within particular species were analysed, limiting the statistical power to conduct more detailed comparisons between the species.

Lactobacilli adhesion to epithelial cells is considered to be one of the most critical characteristics for successful vaginal colonisation (Heinemann *et al.*, 2000; Reid *et al.*, 2001; Gueimonde *et al.*, 2006; Hütt *et al.*, 2016), competitive exclusion of pathogens and immune modulation (Marco *et al.*, 2006). Adhesion factors include mostly proteins, polysaccharides or lipoteichoic acid on the lactobacilli cell surface that mediate host interactions and play important roles in promoting mucosal integrity, pathogen exclusion, as well as immunomodulation via host receptor recognition (Danne & Dramsi, 2012; Kulakauskas *et al.*, 2014). In Chapter 6, it was found that highly adherent lactobacilli isolates induced lower cytokine responses in VK2 cells. Here, proteome profiles were compared between highly adherent and less adherent lactobacilli. It was found that ribonucleoside-triphosphate reductase, an enzyme involved in DNA synthesis and repair, and UPF0342 protein LRC_11170, which is involved in protein-to-protein interactions, were differentially abundant between the two groups. This suggests that these proteins may have additional functions involved with the expression and processing of adhesion proteins or extracellular functions, a phenomenon called moonlighting. In support of this, it has previously been reported that some proteins that have intracellular functions also have additional extracellular functions, as reviewed by Wang *et al.* (Wang *et al.*, 2014). These proteins, including glycolytic enzymes, ribosomal proteins and proteins involved in stress responses, were unexpectedly found to be localised on the outer surface of different lactobacilli strains (Beck *et al.*, 2009; Izquierdo *et al.*, 2009; Saad *et al.*, 2009). Additionally, the elongation factor Tu (EF-Tu) was also unexpectedly isolated from the cell surface of the probiotic species *L. johnsonii* NCC533 and *L. plantarum* 423, where it was shown to mediate the adhesion of the bacteria to human epithelial cells, as well as exclusion of pathogenic bacteria (Granato *et al.*, 1999; Ramiah, van Reenen, & Dicks, 2008). In this Chapter, EF-Tu was not among the significant proteins that correlated with lactobacilli adhesion.

Surface protein aggregation promotion factor, a protein that has been previously associated with lactobacilli adhesion to human epithelial cells (Nishiyama *et al.*, 2015), correlated positively with lactobacilli adhesion to VK2 cells, although this was not upheld after adjusting for species and batch. Previous studies have also identified the following adhesion factors in lactobacilli: mucin binding protein (MacKenzie *et al.*, 2010), aggregation promoting factors, collagen binding proteins, LPXTG-containing proteins and S-layer proteins (Heinemann *et al.*, 2000; Lebeer *et al.*, 2008; Kankainen *et al.*, 2009; Nishiyama *et al.*, 2015). However, although these proteins were expressed in the lactobacilli isolates included in the present study, these proteins did not correlate with lactobacilli adhesion in this analysis.

Lactobacilli are said to protect against pathogens by, amongst other characteristics, production of active metabolites such as lactic acid (Aldunate *et al.*, 2013; Gong *et al.*, 2014). Here the production of D-lactate correlated positively with D-lactate dehydrogenase relative abundance. It has previously been shown that lactic acid may have immunomodulatory properties and inhibits the production of pro-inflammatory cytokines by cervicovaginal epithelial cells (Hearps *et al.*, 2017). Additionally, in Chapter 6 of this book, D-lactate production was negatively correlated with IL-6 production by VK2 cells *in vitro*. In support of these findings, a strong negative correlation was found between D-lactate dehydrogenase relative abundance and inflammatory cytokine responses in this Chapter, further supporting the notion that lactobacilli immunomodulatory properties may be associated with lactic acid production. The mechanisms however remain unknown.

Taken together, these findings show that the differences in the inflammatory properties observed between lactobacilli strains may be associated with differences in their proteome profiles and that the immunomodulation process is likely multifactorial and is not attributed to a single pathway or characteristic. Differences in immunomodulatory properties appear to be linked to the level of metabolic activity, membrane properties, D-lactate dehydrogenase and in turn D-lactate production. Changes in these properties may be due to the adaption of the lactobacilli to different physical environments, as previously proposed (De Angelis *et al.*, 2016), including the high pH environment associated with non-optimal microbiota. This hypothesis is supported by the finding that lactobacilli isolated from women with non-optimal microbiota were found to be more inflammatory *in vitro*. Alternatively, the inherent properties of the lactobacilli may influence the ability of non-optimal bacteria to colonize the FGT. Comparative proteomic analyses may help to identify key genes that play a role in niche or metabolic adaptation, which may be useful in designing strategies for optimal cultivation conditions of probiotic strains to favor improved biotherapeutic characteristics. Furthermore, complex regulatory networks that influence strain specific probiotic traits *in vivo* can be identified to aid in selection of strains with the best health promoting properties.

CHAPTER 8: DISCUSSION

In this dissertation, the biotherapeutic-relevant and immunomodulatory characteristics of cervicovaginal lactobacilli isolates from South African women were evaluated *in vitro* in order to compare the properties of different species and strains that may protect against BV and HIV. Additionally, to evaluate the potential to improve existing commercially available biotherapeutic formulations, the performance of the cervicovaginal lactobacilli was compared to probiotics obtained on the South African market, including *L. casei rhamnosus* and *L. acidophilus*. It was found that *Lactobacillus* characteristics considered to be important for vaginal re-colonization and protection against pathogens, including adhesion to vaginal epithelial cells, culture acidification, D/L-lactate production, growth rates and size, were highly strain-specific, with several novel vaginal *Lactobacillus* isolates performing better than commercial probiotics. Further, it was found that the cervicovaginal *Lactobacillus* isolates suppressed HIV pseudovirus infectivity in a strain-specific manner and resulted in reduced production of several inflammatory cytokines in response to *G. vaginalis* and *P. bivia* when co-cultured with VK2 cells. Interestingly, isolates obtained from women with non-optimal microbiota (Nugent 4-10) induced greater levels of inflammatory cytokine responses and produced less lactic acid than isolates from women with optimal microbiota (Nugent 0-3). Lastly, in Chapter 7, proteome profiles were compared between lactobacilli isolates that induced relatively high versus low levels of inflammatory cytokine production by VK2 cells *in vitro*. It was found that 164 proteins were differentially abundant between the two groups and that isolates inducing lower cytokine responses had a significantly higher relative abundance of membrane-associated cellular components, metabolic biological processes and enzymatic molecular functions compared to isolates that induced higher levels of inflammation.

8.1 Characterisation of vaginal *Lactobacillus* species and strains

Lactobacillus characteristics including growth rates, sizes, adhesion to vaginal epithelial cells, acidification and D/L-lactate production are among the properties thought to be beneficial and important for colonization and persistence in the FGT (Gong *et al*., 2014; Hearps *et al*., 2017; Tyssen *et al*., 2018; Boris *et al*., 1998; Osset *et al*., 2002; Gueimonde *et al*., 2006; Gueimonde & Salminen, 2006; Borgdorff *et al*., 2014; Breshears *et al*., 2015; Matsubara *et al*., 2016). In Chapter

3, these characteristics were evaluated *in vitro* and compared between 64 vaginal *Lactobacillus* isolates, including *L. crispatus*, *L. jensenii*, *L. johnsonii*, *L. mucosae*, *L. plantarum*, *L.ruminis*, *L. salivarius* and *L. vaginalis* species, from the FGT secretions of South African women. Similarly, in Chapter 4, these characteristics were evaluated in a different group of 23 isolates, as well as three probiotics *Lactobacillus* isolates. Although no particular species appeared to markedly outperform the others when the isolates were assigned scores based on all of the characteristics evaluated, of the top ten species of the analyses included in Chapters 3 and 4, 35% were *L. jensenii,* 20% were *L. vaginalis*, while *L. mucosae*, *L. johnsonii, L. crispatus* and the *L. acidophilus* probiotic isolates each comprised 10%. The *L. jensenii* and *L. vaginalis* isolates included in the analysis described in Chapter 3 (including 64 vaginal isolates) produced the most D- and L-lactate, respectively. Similarly, in Chapter 4 (23 isolates), *L. jensenii* and *L. vaginalis* produced the largest amounts of L- and D-lactate, respectively. This suggests that the concentration of lactate in the FGT is highly dependent on the predominant species. When individual strains were compared, it was found that there was large variation at strain level, suggesting that lactate concentrations in the FGT are also dependent on the lactobacilli strains. Similar to previous findings (O'Hanlon *et al.*, 2013), it was found that *Lactobacillus* culture pH correlated negatively with lactic acid production by the lactobacilli, supporting the notion that lactate production by lactobacilli plays a critical role in acidification in the FGT. *L. jensenii* isolates were the most adherent of the clinical isolates, while *L. crispatus* and *L. salivarius* isolates in Chapters 3 and 4 grew most rapidly.

Although an *L. crispatus*-dominated vaginal microbiome is considered to be particularly optimal, as this species has been associated with stability of the vaginal microbiota (Boskey *et al.*, 1999; Pendharkar *et al.*, 2013; Verstraelen *et al.*, 2009), reduced risk of HIV acquisition (Doerflinger *et al.*, 2014; Gosmann *et al.*, 2017), as well as reduced risk of conversion from optimal to non-optimal vaginal microbiota (Boskey *et al.*, 1999; Pendharkar *et al.*, 2013; Verstraelen *et al.*, 2009), other *Lactobacillus* species, most notably *L. jensenii*, performed as well, if not better than the *L. crispatus* isolates included in this *in vitro* study. *L. crispatus* isolates were mostly poorly adherent relative to the species evaluated, although the isolates of this species did produce significant amounts of lactate and exhibited rapid growth. *L. crispatus* dominance is rare in African women (Anahtar *et al.*, 2015; Klatt *et al.*, 2017; Lennard *et al.*, 2017) and differences in the properties of *L. crispatus* strains from African versus American and European women may be a contributing factor. Key studies conducted in South African women that demonstrated reduced levels of FGT inflammation and HIV risk in women with non-*iners Lactobacillus* dominance did not distinguish between different non-*iners Lactobacillus* species (Anahtar *et al.*, 2015; Gosmann *et al.*, 2017). Another study in South African women found that an operational taxonomic unit annotated as *L. johnsonii/gasseri* was more important for prediction of FGT inflammation than *L. crispatus/acidophilus* (Lennard *et al.*, 2017). In the present study, it was found that, while there was an approximately equal distribution of *L. crispatus* isolates from women with optimal versus non-optimal microbiota, a greater number of *L. jensenii* were isolated from women with optimal microbiota. In support, a previous study similarly identified an almost equal distribution in *L. crispatus* isolates obtained from South African women with and without BV, while significantly fewer *L. jensenii* isolates were obtained from women with BV relative to those without BV (Damelin *et al.*, 2011). Thus, the relative health benefits of *L. crispatus* versus other non-*iners* lactobacilli in African women remain unclear and future studies to compare particular species from women of different ethnicities or residing in different geographical locations would be highly informative.

Interestingly, when beneficial characteristics were compared between lactobacilli isolates from women with optimal versus non-optimal microbiota, it was found that isolates that were obtained from women with non-optimal microbiota produced significantly lower amounts of D-lactate and lactic acid, which may reflect an inability to competitively exclude pathogenic bacteria in the FGT. These differences in lactic acid production may be a result of the differences in species distribution between women with optimal versus non-optimal microbiota or, alternatively, due to *Lactobacillus* adaption to the high pH environment associated with non-optimal microbiota. In support, previous studies have demonstrated modifications of *Lactobacillus* proteins belonging to various functional categories in order to adapt to different environmental niches or stresses (Bove *et al.*, 2012; De Angelis *et al.*, 2016; Siragusa *et al.*, 2014; Wang *et al.*, 2018). Overall in this dissertation, there was a large variation in characteristics both within and between species that corresponds to previous findings (Samuel *et al.*, 2016; Mclean *et al.*, 2000; Pino *et al.*, 2019). These findings suggest that, although lactobacilli have been shown to have protective properties, different *Lactobacillus* strains may vary in their capacity to protect the FGT from colonisation by bacterial and viral pathogens (Osset *et al.*, 2001; Verstraelen *et al.*, 2009). This highlights the importance of thoroughly screening vaginal isolates for the best probiotic candidates.

8.2 Comparison of biotherapeutic-relevant characteristics between vaginal *Lactobacillus* isolates and probiotics

To evaluate the potential to improve existing probiotics for treatment of BV, the biotherapeutic-relevant properties of commercial probiotics found on the South African market were compared to 23 vaginal *Lactobacillus* isolates. All of the isolates and commercial probiotics analysed here produced detectable amounts of D-lactate and varying concentrations of L-lactate. When compared to the probiotic *Lactobacillus* isolates, the vaginal lactobacilli produced more lactic acid both in co-culture with Ca Ski cells and on their own, suggesting that the probiotics may be less protective than the vaginal lactobacilli, as lactic acid production is considered to be one of the most important mechanisms underlying the protective effect of lactobacilli (Witkin *et al.*, 2013). Interestingly, both the *L. acidophilus* tablet and *L. casei rhamnosus* did not produce detectable amounts of L-lactate in culture. Following a 24 hour incubation period in MRS broth, the clinical lactobacilli and probiotic isolates analysed here were able to acidify the culture medium to a range (3.7-5.6) that closely matched that seen in *Lactobacillus*-dominated FGTs (3.2-4.5) (O'Hanlon *et al.*, 2013). BV is associated with an elevated vaginal pH as vaginal lactobacilli are lost while an overgrowth of diverse bacteria including non-optimal microbiota such as *G. vaginalis*, *Atopobium*, and *P. bivia* occurs (Ravel *et al.*, 2011). Interestingly, the *L. casei rhamnosus* and *L. acidophilus* probiotics acidified the culture medium the most compared to the vaginal isolates, despite producing relatively little lactic acid. This suggests the production of organic acids other than lactic acid such as acetic, propionic, butyric, formic, citric, succinic and glutamic acids which are also produced by lactobacilli species (Özcelik *et al.*, 2016; Zalán *et al.*, 2010). One of the *L. acidophilus* probiotic isolates was the most adherent, although the differences observed between species analysed were not statistically significant, due to both the wide variation in the properties of individual strains of each species, as well as the small sample sizes. The differences in the protective characteristics between these commercial probiotics, as well as vaginal lactobacilli strains and species, that were observed in this and previous studies (Osset et al., 2001; Sanders, 2008) may explain the substantial heterogeneity in efficacy that has been observed during clinical trials to evaluate the efficacy of probiotic administration for BV treatment (Bisanz *et al.*, 2014; Bohbot *et al.*, 2018; Bradshaw *et al.*, 2012; Hemalatha *et al.*, 2012; Ling *et al.*, 2013; Machado *et al.*, 2016; Mastromarino *et al.*, 2009; Rapisarda *et al.*, 2018; Verdenelli *et al.*, 2016).

Overall the findings in Chapter 4 showed that some vaginal isolates, including three *L. jensenii* strains, performed better than isolates obtained from the commercial probiotics analysed here, with variation in probiotic-relevant characteristics both between lactobacilli strains and species. Additionally the lactobacilli isolated from the commercial probiotics were not among the species isolated from the FGTs of the women described in Chapter 4, as well as Chapter 3. Taken together, these findings support the importance of thoroughly evaluating candidate probiotics to improve the formulations available on the South African market.

8.3 Immunomodulatory properties of vaginal *Lactobacillus* isolates

In Chapter 6, *in vitro* systems were used to evaluate the immunomodulatory capabilities of the vaginal *Lactobacillus* isolates by measuring the concentrations of proinflammatory cytokines secreted by vaginal epithelial (VK2) cells in response to vaginal *Lactobacillus* isolates, and *G. vaginalis* and *P. bivia* ATCC reference strains. Interestingly, in addition to producing less lactic acid as described above, isolates from women with non-optimal microbiota induced greater inflammatory cytokine responses in VK2 cells than isolates from women with optimal microbiota. When co-cultured with *G. vaginalis* the majority of the lactobacilli significantly suppressed overall inflammatory responses to *G. vaginalis* as previously shown (Rose *et al.*, 2012; Santos *et al.*, 2018; Chetwin *et al.*, 2019), causing significant decreases in IL-6 and IL-8, as well as non-significant decreases in IP-10, MIP-1α, MIP-1β and MIP-3α relative to *G. vaginalis*-only cultures. However, pre-incubation with lactobacilli also resulted in significantly elevated IL-1α and IL-1β responses. Although this was unexpected, it suggests that co-culturing vaginal epithelial cells with both lactobacilli and *G. vaginalis* had an additive effect on the IL-1 pathway and that the production of the other cytokines assessed may be regulated through alternative pathways. Furthermore, the IL-1 pathway is regulated both post-transcriptionally and translationally and involves complex regulated checkpoints compared to other cytokine systems (Carta *et al.*, 2013; Mayer-Barber & Yan, 2017), which may explain the difference in expression of IL-1 compared to other cytokines evaluated here. Most importantly, the majority of cytokines, including key chemokines that specifically recruit target cells for HIV infection (Wira *et al.*, 2010), were suppressed by the lactobacilli and cumulative median cytokine levels were lower following pre-incubation with lactobacilli compared to *G. vaginalis* only cultures. This suggests that lactobacilli may decrease HIV acquisition risk by reducing inflammatory cytokine production in the FGT.

On the other hand, non-significant upregulation of the majority of the cytokines evaluated, including MIP-1α, MIP-1β, MIP-3α, IL-6, IL-1α and IL-8, was observed following incubation with *P. bivia*. This was not expected, as this species has been associated with high levels of inflammatory cytokines *in vivo* (Jousimies–Somer, 1997; Hummelen *et al.*, 2010). However, it has previously been suggested that the capacity to induce a weak pro-inflammatory cytokine response by *P. bivia* strains may be a virulence factor to evade the immune system and establish a productive infection (Strömbeck *et al.*, 2007). A previous study further showed that the same *P. bivia* ATCC reference strain as the one evaluated in the present study, did not induce significant inflammatory responses when co-cultured with vaginal epithelial cells, although changes in antimicrobial peptides and mucin expression were observed, suggesting that *P. bivia* may still compromise the epithelial barrier function without induction of significant inflammatory responses (Doerflinger *et al.*, 2014). It is thus possible that the strain used in this dissertation has a less inflammatory nature compared to other *P. bivia* strains. In support of this, it has previously been shown that when different *P. bivia* strains were each co-cultured with HeLa cells, some of the strains were only able to induce weak proinflammatory cytokine responses, suggesting that the capacity to induce cytokine responses may be strain specific (Strömbeck *et al.*, 2007). Additionally, the vaginal epithelial cells used in this study express very little toll-like receptor (TLR)-4 (Fichorova *et al.*, 2002; Fazeli *et al.*, 2005), which recognizes lipopolysaccharide (LPS) in the cell walls of Gram negative bacteria including *P. bivia* (Zariffard *et al.*, 2005; Janssens & Beyaert, 2003; Tobita *et al.*, 2016). Therefore *P. bivia* may fail to induce pattern recognition receptor signaling in this model.

Interestingly, only *L. crispatus* isolates markedly suppressed cytokine production that was induced in response to *P. bivia*, while *L. jensenii* and *L. mucosae* isolates were only able to suppress IP-10 responses. These findings were similar to a previous study which showed that co-culturing *P. bivia* with vaginal lactobacilli reduced the viability of *P. bivia* with varying levels of efficacy between species (Atassi *et al.*, 2006). In this dissertation, this may also reflect that there may have been a varying abundance of viable *P. bivia* between the co-cultures after co-incubation with lactobacilli isolates. This may explain the variation in level of inflammatory cytokine suppression observed between the different lactobacilli species as the level of cytokine induction by *P. bivia* strains has been shown to be dependent on the concentration of the strain in culture (Strömbeck *et al.*, 2007). These findings suggest that commensals and pathogens may not be as distinct regarding inflammatory profiles (Doerflinger *et al.*, 2014). Additionally, these findings suggest that lactobacilli possess immunomodulatory properties and that it is critical to obtain *Lactobacillus* isolates from women with optimal microbiota and to fully characterise the inflammatory properties of potential vaginal probiotics.

8.4 Immunomodulatory mechanisms of *Lactobacillus* isolates

When possible mechanisms underlying the immunomodulatory properties of the *Lactobacillus* isolates were investigated, it was found that D-lactate production by the lactobacilli was inversely associated with IL-6 production in the *Lactobacillus/G.vaginalis* co-cultures. Interestingly, the majority of differentially expressed proteins were under-represented in lactobacilli that induced high inflammatory cytokine responses by VK2 cells. Under-represented GOs included membrane-associated cellular components, metabolic biological processes and enzymatic and transmembrane transport molecular functions. Borgdorff *et al.* showed that protein expression may be significantly downregulated at pH ranges associated with non-optimal microbiomes, possibly as a result of a decline in metabolic activity in the lactobacilli (Hanneke Borgdorff *et al.*, 2016). A decline in metabolic activity may result in reduced production of lactic acid, which in turn suppresses inflammatory responses. In support, a strong negative correlation was found between D-lactate dehydrogenase relative abundance, D-lactate production and inflammatory cytokine responses. Additionally, Hearps *et al.* (2017) previously demonstrated that lactic acid suppressed inflammatory cytokine production in *in vitro* cervicovaginal epithelial cell cultures.

It was additionally found that removing unbound lactobacilli and the culture supernatant prior to addition of *G. vaginalis* reduced the level of suppression of inflammatory responses, although cytokine downregulation was still observed. This suggests that both the production of metabolites and direct interaction between the lactobacilli and epithelial cells are important for immunomodulation. In line with this, in addition to D-lactate production, adhesion of lactobacilli to vaginal epithelial cells was inversely associated with cytokine responses. Moreover, the overabundance of membrane cellular components and proteins involved with transmembrane transport in less inflammatory isolates suggests that the majority of the differentially abundant proteins were localised to the membrane. This in turn suggests that interaction between the *Lactobacillus* membrane and host cells, as well as membrane transport systems, play an important role in modulating inflammatory responses as has previously been reported in studies of gastrointestinal lactobacilli (Kulakauskas & Chapot-Chartier, 2014). To further investigate the relationships between membrane components, adhesion and inflammation, proteome profiles were also compared between highly adherent and weakly adherent lactobacilli isolates. Surface protein aggregation promotion factor showed a trend towards a positive correlation with lactobacilli adhesion to VK2 cells while ribonucleoside-triphosphate reductase, an enzyme involved with DNA synthesis and repair, and UPF0342 protein LRC_11170 were differentially abundant between the two groups. This suggests that these proteins may have additional functions involved with the expression and processing of adhesion proteins or extracellular functions, a phenomenon called moonlighting (Dhanani & Bagchi, 2013; Wang *et al.*, 2014; Waśko *et al.*, 2014)

Taken together these findings suggest that the reduction in cytokine secretion observed in the *Lactobacillus/G.vaginalis* co-cultures may be due to competitive inhibition of *G. vaginalis* interaction with the vaginal epithelial cells, as well as an effect of metabolites including lactic acid being secreted by the lactobacilli. It has also been previously reported that vaginal lactobacilli reduce the expression of TLR4, which recognizes LPS in the cell walls of Gram negative bacteria (Zariffard *et al.*, 2005; Janssens & Beyaert, 2003; Tobita *et al.*, 2016). Although it seems that *G. vaginalis* does not express LPS (Sadhu *et al.*, 1989; Marin *et al.*, 2018) and vaginal epithelial cells express little TLR4 (Fichorova *et al.*, 2002; Fazeli *et al.*, 2005), lactobacilli may suppress cytokine responses to *G. vaginalis* by reducing the production of other pattern recognition receptors. The mechanism by which lactic acid may alter inflammatory responses is unknown. However, it was previously shown that lactic acid induced upregulated anti-inflammatory IL-1RA expression by cervicovaginal epithelial cells (Hearps *et al.*, 2017), which may in turn suppress the IL-1 pathway by binding to cell surface IL-1 receptor and therefore preventing the binding of IL-1α and IL-1β

cytokines (Yazdi & Goreschi, 2016). In this dissertation significant levels of IL-1RA were detected in the *Lactobacillus*-only cultures (including 64 isolates). Although IL-1RA production was not evaluated in the *Lactobacillus/G.vaginalis* co-cultures, it was found that the production of both IL-1α and IL-1β were increased in response to co-culture with lactobacilli and *G. vaginalis* compared to *G. vaginalis* only stimulation. Similarly, Hearps *et al.* (2017) found that IL-1β production was significantly increased following lactic acid treatment. Taken together, these findings suggest that markedly increased production of IL-1RA may mitigate the downstream inflammatory effects of increased IL-1α and IL-1β production.

In Chapter 6, lactobacilli isolated from women with non-optimal microbiota were more inflammatory and produced less lactic acid than those isolated from women with optimal microbiota. These findings suggest that high vaginal pH in women with non-optimal microbiota may result in the adaption of *Lactobacillus* species, involving reduced metabolic activity and lactic acid production, as well as adhesion capacity, that in turn hinders the immunomodulatory abilities of these isolates. Taken together, these findings show that the immunomodulation process is likely multifactorial and is not attributed to a single pathway or characteristic.

8.5 Modulation of HIV pseudovirus infectivity by *Lactobacillus* isolates

In Chapter 5, it was found that lactobacilli-conditioned culture medium inhibited HIV pseudovirus infectivity in a strain-specific manner, with *L. crispatus*-conditioned and *L. vaginalis*-conditioned culture medium conferring the greatest degree of inhibition. In the experiment, abiotic *Lactobacillus* culture medium was added to TZM-bl cells in the presence of the HIV pseudovirus, suggesting that the inhibition may have been due to metabolites produced by the lactobacilli (Aldunate *et al.*, 2015, 2013; Hearps *et al.*, 2017; Tyssen *et al.*, 2018). Similarly, a previous study showed that incubation of HIV-1 in lactobacilli-conditioned medium significantly inhibited viral infectivity, as well as replication, in human tissues *ex vivo* and inhibition correlated with lactic acid concentration (Palomino *et al.*, 2017). However, in the present study, while lactic acid concentration was not associated with infectivity, culture pH was inversely correlated with infectivity. The lack of association between lactic acid suggests that the lactobacilli culture supernatant may have a direct virucidal effect on the HIV pseudovirus resulting in reduced infectivity as previously suggested (Palomino *et al.*, 2017). Though the sample size in Chapter 5 was small, there was no significant difference between *Lactobacillus* isolates from women with optimal microbiota versus non-optimal microbiota. This may have been due to the fact that there were no differences in culture acidification between the isolates since virucidal activity has been shown in this and previous studies to be pH-dependent (Aldunate *et al.*, 2013; Tyssen *et al.*, 2018). HIV infectivity was also associated with IL-1α and IL-1β production by VK2 cells in response to the same isolates. IL-1 is associated with activation of NF-Kβ which promotes HIV viral replication (Muzio *et al.*, 1998; Osborn *et al.*, 1989; Wira *et al.*, 2005), suggesting that an upregulation of these cytokines in the FGT may increase HIV acquisition risk as has previously been reported (Nazli *et al.*, 2010; Osborn *et al.*, 1989; Wira *et al.*, 2005). However, a limitation of this study was that HIV pseudovirus entry was evaluated in TZM-bl cells *in vitro* in a different system to the cytokine experiments.

Overall, these findings suggest that the presence of *Lactobacillus* species in the FGT may protect against HIV infection in a species-specific manner, as previously reported (Tyssen *et al.*, 2018). However, the variation observed between different strains may also suggest that the level of protection is strain-specific of which culture pH seem to play a major role. The findings in Chapter 5 suggest that the HIV infectivity assay may be used to screen for the best lactobacilli isolates that strongly suppress HIV infectivity for use in biotherapeutics for HIV prevention in women.

8.6 Conclusion

In summary, since several vaginal lactobacilli performed better than probiotic lactobacilli, these findings demonstrate the potential to improve the current probiotics with formulations that include *Lactobacillus* species that predominate in an optimal FGT in order to improve BV treatment outcomes. Another key finding of this study was the large amount of variation in protective characteristics both between and within vaginal lactobacilli species. The results both provide a better understanding of the immunomodulatory properties of *Lactobacillus* species, as well as the underlying mechanisms, identifying possible targets for further exploration as biotherapeutics applications. The differences in lactobacilli isolated from women with optimal versus non-optimal microbiota may be the result of the adaptation of the lactobacilli to different physical environments. Alternatively, the inherent characteristics of the lactobacilli may have influenced the ability of pathogenic bacteria to colonize the FGT. Longitudinal proteomic analyses may help to identify important protein pathways that play key roles in niche adaptation which may be useful in designing strategies for optimal cultivation conditions of probiotic candidates. Furthermore, gene expression analyses would be useful to determine the inflammatory signaling pathways that are modulated by lactobacilli. This study emphasizes the functional diversity of the vaginal microbiome that exists at the strain level that markedly influences both biotherapeutic potential and inflammatory responses, highlighting the importance of rigorous screening of lactobacilli isolates prior to probiotic development.

REFERENCES

Abbas, A. K., Lichtman, A. H., & Pillai, S. (2016). Functions and disorders of the immune system. *Basic Immunology*, 147–168.

Abdool Karim, Q., Abdool Karim, S., Frohlich, J. A., Grobler, A. C., Baxter, C., Mansoor, L. E., … Taylor, D. (2010). Effectiveness and safety of tenofovir gel, an antiretroviral microbicide, for the prevention of HIV infection in women. *Science*, *329*(AUG), 988–993.

Al-Naseri, A., Bowman, J. P., Wilson, R., Nilsson, R. E., & Britz, M. L. (2013). Impact of lactose starvation on the physiology of *Lactobacillus casei* GCRL163 in the presence or absence of Tween 80. *Journal of Proteome Research*, *12*(11), 5313-5322.

Al Kassaa, I., Hober, D., Hamze, M., Chihib, N. E., & Drider, D. (2014). Antiviral potential of lactic acid bacteria and their bacteriocins. *Probiotics and Antimicrobial Proteins*, *6*(3–4), 177–185.

Alander, M., Satokari, R., Korpela, R., Vilpponen-salmela, T., Mattila-sandholm, T., & Wright, A. Von. (1999). Persistence of colonization of human colonic mucosa by a probiotic strain, *Lactobacillus rhamnosus* GG, after oral consumption persistence of colonization of human colonic mucosa by a probiotic strain , *Lactobacillus rhamnosus* GG , after oral consumption. *Applied and Environmental Microbiology*, *65*(1), 351–354.

Aldunate, M., Srbinovski, D., Hearps, A. C., Latham, C. F., Ramsland, P. A., Gugasyan, R., … Tachedjian, G. (2015). Antimicrobial and immune modulatory effects of lactic acid and short chain fatty acids produced by vaginal microbiota associated with eubiosis and bacterial vaginosis. *Frontiers in Physiology*, *6*(JUN), 1–23.

Aldunate, M., Tyssen, D., Johnson, A., Zakir, T., Sonza, S., Moench, T., … Tachedjian, G. (2013). Vaginal concentrations of lactic acid potently inactivate HIV. *Journal of Antimicrobial Chemotherapy*, *68*(9), 2015–2025.

Allsworth, J. E., Lewis, V. A., & Peipert, J. F. (2008). Viral sexually transmitted infections and bacterial vaginosis: 2001-2004 national health and nutrition examination survey data. *Sexually Transmitted Diseases*, *35*(9), 791–796.

Allsworth, J. E., & Peipert, J. F. (2007b). Prevalence of bacterial vaginosis: 2001-2004 National Health and Nutrition Examination Survey data. *Obstetrics and Gynecology*, *109*(1), 114–120.

Amjadi, F., Salehi, E., Mehdizadeh, M., & Aflatoonian, R. (2014). Role of the innate immunity in female reproductive tract. *Advanced Biomedical Research*, *3*, 1.

Amor, K. Ben, Breeuwer, P., Verbaarschot, P., Rombouts, F. M., Akkermans, A. D. L., Vos, W. M. De, & Abee, T. (2002). Multiparametric flow cytometry and cell sorting for the assessment of viable injured and dead cells. *Applied and Environmental Microbiology*, *68*(11), 5209–5216.

Amsel, R., Totten, P. A., Spiegel, C. A., Chen, K. C. S., Eschenbach, D., & Holmes, K. K. (1983). Nonspecific vaginitis: Diagnostic criteria and microbial and epidemiologic associations. *The American Journal of Medicine*, *74*(1), 14–22.

Anahtar, M N, Byrne, E. H., Doherty, K. E., Bowman, B. A., Yamamoto, H. S., Soumillon, M., … Sabatini, M. E. (2015). Cervicovaginal bacteria are a major modulator of host inflammatory responses in the female genital tract. *Immunity*, *42*, 965–976.

Anahtar, Melis N., Gootenberg, D. B., Mitchell, C. M., & Kwon, D. S. (2018). Cervicovaginal microbiota and reproductive health: The virtue of simplicity. *Cell Host and Microbe*, *23*(2), 159–168.

Anderson, A. C., Karygianni, L., Hellwig, E., Al-Ahmad, A., Sanunu, M., Schneider, C., & Clad, A. (2014). Rapid species-level identification of vaginal and oral lactobacilli using MALDI-

TOF MS analysis and 16S rDNA sequencing. *Biomed Central Microbiology*, *14*(1), 1–9.

Anderson, D., Politch, J. A., & Pudney, J. (2011). HIV Infection and immune defense of the penis. *American Journal of Reproductive Immunology*, *65*(3), 220–229.

Andreu, A., Stapleton, A. E., Fennell, C. L., Hillier, S. L., & Stamm, W. E. (1995). Hemagglutination, adherence, and surface properties of vaginal *Lactobacillus* species. *Journal of Infectious Diseases*, *171*(5), 1237–1243.

Antonio, M. A. D., Meyn, L. A., Murray, P. J., Busse, B., & Hillier, S. L. (2009). Vaginal colonization by probiotic *Lactobacillus crispatus* CTV-05 is decreased by sexual activity and endogenous lactobacilli . *The Journal of Infectious Diseases*, *199*(10), 1506–1513.

Antonio, M. A., Hawes, S. E., & Hillier, S. L. (1999). The identification of vaginal *Lactobacillus* species and the demographic and microbiologic characteristics of women colonised by these species. *Journal of Infectious Diseases*, 180(6), 1950–1956.

Anukam, K. C. . b d, Osazuwa, E. O. ., Ahonkhai, I. ., & Reid, G. . c. (2005). 16S rRNA gene sequence and phylogenetic tree of *Lactobacillus* species from the vagina of healthy Nigerian women. *African Journal of Biotechnology*, *4*(11), 1222–1227.

Anukam, K. C., Osazuwa, E., Osemene, G. I., Ehigiagbe, F., Bruce, A. W., & Reid, G. (2006). Clinical study comparing probiotic *Lactobacillus* GR-1 and RC-14 with metronidazole vaginal gel to treat symptomatic bacterial vaginosis. *Microbes and Infection*, *8*(12–13), 2772–2776.

Anukam, K., Osazuwa, E., Ahonkhai, I., Ngwu, M., Osemene, G., Bruce, A. W., & Reid, G. (2006). Augmentation of antimicrobial metronidazole therapy of bacterial vaginosis with oral probiotic *Lactobacillus rhamnosus* GR-1 and *Lactobacillus reuteri* RC-14: randomized, double-blind, placebo controlled trial. *Microbes and Infection*, *8*(6), 1450–1454.

Anukam, K., Duru, M., Eze, C., Egharevba, J., Aiyebelehin, A., Bruce, A., & Reid, G. (2009). Oral use of probiotics as an adjunctive therapy to fluconazole in the treatment of yeast vaginitis: A study of nigerian women in an outdoor clinic. *Microbial Ecology in Health and Disease*, *21*(2), 72–77.

Arena, M. P., Capozzi, V., Russo, P., Drider, D., Spano, G., & Fiocco, D. (2018). Immunobiosis and probiosis: antimicrobial activity of lactic acid bacteria with a focus on their antiviral and antifungal properties. *Applied Microbiology and Biotechnology*, *102*(23), 9949–9958.

Arena, M. P., Elmastour, F., Sane, F., Drider, D., Fiocco, D., Spano, G., & Hober, D. (2018). Inhibition of coxsackievirus B4 by *Lactobacillus plantarum*. *Microbiological Research*, *210*(December), 59–64.

Arnold, K. B., Burgener, A., Birse, K., Romas, L., Dunphy, L. J., Shahabi, K., … McKinnon, L. R. (2016). Increased levels of inflammatory cytokines in the female reproductive tract are associated with altered expression of proteases, mucosal barrier proteins, and an influx of HIV-susceptible target cells. *Mucosal Immunology*, *9*(1), 194–205.

Aroutcheva, A., Gariti, D., Simon, M., Shott, S., Faro, J., Simoes, J. A., … Faro, S. (2001). Defense factors of vaginal lactobacilli. *American Journal of Obstetrics and Gynecology*, *185*(2), 375–379.

Atashili, J., Poole, C., Ndumbe, P. M., Adimora, A. A., & Smith, J. S. (2008). Bacterial vaginosis and HIV acquisition: A meta-analysis of published studies. *Aids*, *22*(12), 1493–1501.

Atassi, F., Brassart, D., Grob, P., Graf, F., & Servin, A. L. (2006). *Lactobacillus* strains isolated from the vaginal microbiota of healthy women inhibit *Prevotella bivia* and *Gardnerella vaginalis* in coculture and cell culture. *FEMS Immunology and Medical Microbiology*, *48*(3), 424–432.

Atujuna, M., Newman, P. A., Wallace, M., Eluhu, M., Rubincam, C., Brown, B., & Bekker, L. G. (2018). Contexts of vulnerability and the acceptability of new biomedical HIV prevention technologies among key populations in South Africa: A qualitative study. *PLoS one*, *13*(2), 1–17.

Barnabas, S. L., Dabee, S., Passmore, J.-A. S., Jaspan, H. B., Lewis, D. A., Jaumdally, S. Z., Bekker, L.-G. (2017). Converging epidemics of sexually transmitted infections and bacterial vaginosis in southern African female adolescents at risk of HIV. *International Journal of STD & AIDS*, *29*(6), 531–539.

Barrons, R., & Tassone, D. (2008). Use of *Lactobacillus* probiotics for bacterial genitourinary infections in women: a review. *Clinical Therapeutics*, 30(3), 453-468.

Beck, H. C., Madsen, S. M., Glenting, J., Petersen, J., Israelsen, H., Nørrelykke, M. R., … Hansen, A. M. (2009). Proteomic analysis of cell surface-associated proteins from probiotic *Lactobacillus plantarum*. *FEMS Microbiology Letters*, *297*(1), 61–66.

Beigi, R. H., Austin, M. N., Meyn, L. A., Krohn, M. A., & Hillier, S. L. (2004). Antimicrobial resistance associated with the treatment of bacterial vaginosis. *American Journal of Obstetrics and Gynecology*, *191*(4), 1124–1129.

Berard, A. R., Perner, M., Mutch, S., Farr Zuend, C., McQueen, P., & Burgener, A. D. (2018). Understanding mucosal and microbial functionality of the female reproductive tract by metaproteomics: Implications for HIV transmission. *American Journal of Reproductive Immunology*, *80*(2).

Bisanz, J. E., Seney, S., McMillan, A., Vongsa, R., Koenig, D., Wong, L., Reid, G. (2014). A systems biology approach investigating the effect of probiotics on the vaginal microbiome and host responses in a double blind, placebo-controlled clinical trial of post-menopausal women. *PLOS ONE*, *9*(8), e104511.

Bohbot, J. M., Daraï, E., Bretelle, F., Brami, G., Daniel, C., & Cardot, J. M. (2018). Efficacy and safety of vaginally administered lyophilized *Lactobacillus crispatus* IP 174178 in the prevention of bacterial vaginosis recurrence. *Journal of Gynecology Obstetrics and Human Reproduction*, *47*(2), 81–86.

Borgdorff, H, Gautam, R., Armstrong, S., Xia, D., Ndayisaba, G., van Teijlingen, N., … van de Wijgert, J. (2015). Cervicovaginal microbiome dysbiosis is associated with proteome changes related to alterations of the cervicovaginal mucosal barrier. *Sexually Transmitted Infections*, *91*(Suppl 2), A54.1-A54.

Borgdorff, Hanneke, Armstrong, S. D., Tytgat, H. L. P., Xia, D., Ndayisaba, G. F., Wastling, J. M., & Van De Wijgert, J. H. H. M. (2016). Unique insights in the cervicovaginal *Lactobacillus iners* and *L. crispatus* proteomes and their associations with microbiota dysbiosis. *PLoS ONE*, *11*(3), 1–14.

Borgdorff, Hanneke, Tsivtsivadze, E., Verhelst, R., Marzorati, M., Jurriaans, S., Ndayisaba, G. F., … Van De Wijgert, J. H. H. M. (2014). *Lactobacillus*-dominated cervicovaginal microbiota associated with reduced HIV/STI prevalence and genital HIV viral load in african women. *ISME Journal*, *8*(9), 1781–1793.

Boris, Soledad, & Barbés, C. (2000). Role played by lactobacilli in controlling the population of vaginal pathogens. *Microbes and Infection*, *2*(5), 543–546.

Boris, Soledad, Suárez, J. E., Vázquez, F., & Barbés, C. (1998). Adherence of human vaginal lactobacilli to vaginal epithelial cells and interaction with uropathogens. *Infection and Immunity*, *66*(5), 1985–1989.

Borish, L. C., & Steinke, J. W. (2003). 2. Cytokines and chemokines. *Journal of Allergy and*

Clinical Immunology, *111*(2 SUPPL. 2), 460–475.

Boskey, E. R., Cone, R. A., Whaley, K. J., & Moench, T. R. (2001). Origins of vaginal acidity: high D/L lactate ratio is consistent with bacteria being the primary source. *Human Reproduction*, *16*(9), 1809–1813.

Boskey, E. R., Telsch, K. M., Whaley, K. J., Moench, T. R., & Cone, R. A. (1999). Acid production by vaginal flora in vitro is consistent with the rate and extent of vaginal acidification. *Infection and Immunity*, *67*(10), 5170–5175.

Bouhnik, Y., Flourié, B., D'Agay-Abensour, L., Pochart, P., Gramet, G., Durand, M., & Rambaud, J.-C. (1997). Administration of transgalacto-oligosaccharides increases fecal bifidobacteria and modifies colonic fermentation metabolism in healthy humans. *The Journal of Nutrition*, *127*(3), 444–448.

Bove, C. G., De Angelis, M., Gatti, M., Calasso, M., Neviani, E., & Gobbetti, M. (2012). Metabolic and proteomic adaptation of *Lactobacillus rhamnosus* strains during growth under cheese-like environmental conditions compared to de Man Rogosa and Sharpe medium. *Proteomics*, *12*(21), 3206–3218.

Bradshaw, C. S., Morton, A. N., Hocking, J., Garland, S. M., Morris, M. B., Moss, L. M., … Fairley, C. K. (2006). High recurrence rates of bacterial vaginosis over the course of 12 months after oral metronidazole therapy and factors associated with recurrence. *The Journal of Infectious Diseases*, *193*(11), 1478–1486.

Bradshaw, C. S., Pirotta, M., de Guingand, D., Hocking, J. S., Morton, A. N., Garland, S. M., … Fairley, C. K. (2012). Efficacy of oral metronidazole with vaginal clindamycin or vaginal probiotic for bacterial vaginosis: Randomised placebo-controlled double-blind trial. *PLoS one*, *7*(4), 1–10.

Breshears, L. M., Edwards, V. L., Ravel, J., & Peterson, M. L. (2015). *Lactobacillus crispatus* inhibits growth of *Gardnerella vaginalis* and *Neisseria gonorrhoeae* on a porcine vaginal mucosa model. *BMC Microbiology*, *15*(1), 1–12.

Brooks, J. P., Edwards, D. J., Blithe, D. L., Fettweis, J. M., Serrano, M. G., Sheth, N. U., … Jefferson, K. K. (2017). Effects of combined oral contraceptives, depot medroxyprogesterone acetate and the levonorgestrel-releasing intrauterine system on the vaginal microbiome. *Contraception*, *95*(4), 405–413.

Brotman, R. M. (2011). Vaginal microbiome and sexually transmitted infections : an epidemiologic perspective, *121*(12), 4610–4617.

Brotman, R. M., Klebanoff, M. A., Nansel, T. R., Yu, K. F., Andrews, W. W., Zhang, J., & Schwebke, J. R. (2010). Bacterial vaginosis assessed by Gram stain and diminished colonization resistance to incident gonococcal, chlamydial, and trichomonal genital infection. *Journal of Infectious Diseases*, *202*(12), 1907–1915.

Brotman, R. M., Ravel, J., Cone, R. A., & Zenilman, J. M. (2010). Rapid fluctuation of the vaginal microbiota measured by Gram stain analysis. *Sexually Transmitted Infections*, *86*(4), 297–302.

Buck, L. B. ., Altermann, E., Svingerud, T., & Klaenhammer, T. R. (2005). Functional analysis of adhesion factors and signaling mechanisms in *Lactobacillus acidophilus*. *Applied and Environmental Microbiology*, *71*(12), 8344–8351.

Burton, J. P., Cadieux, P. A., & Reid, G. (2003). Improved understanding of the bacterial vaginal microbiota of women before and after probiotic instillation. *Applied and Environmental Microbiology*, *69*(1), 97 – 101.

Burton, J. P., & Reid, G. (2002). Evaluation of the bacterial vaginal flora of 20 postmenopausal women by direct (Nugent Score) and molecular (polymerase chain reaction and denaturing gradient gel electrophoresis) techniques. *The Journal of Infectious Diseases*, *186*(12), 1770–1780.

Cai, H., Thompson, R., Budinich, M. F., Broadbent, J. R., & Steele, J. L. (2009). Genome sequence and comparative genome analysis of *Lactobacillus casei*: Insights into their niche-associated evolution. *Genome Biology and Evolution*, *1*(2006), 239–257.

Cai, T., Mazzoli, S., Mondaini, N., Meacci, F., Nesi, G., D'Elia, C., … Bartoletti, R. (2012). The role of asymptomatic bacteriuria in young women with recurrent urinary tract infections: To treat or not to treat? *Clinical Infectious Diseases*, *55*(6), 771–777.

Carta, S., Lavieri, R., & Rubartelli, A. (2013). Different members of the IL-1 family come out in different ways: DAMPs vs. cytokines? *Frontiers in Immunology*, *4*(MAY), 1–9.

Castro, J., Martins, A. P., Rodrigues, M. E., & Cerca, N. (2018). *Lactobacillus crispatus* represses vaginolysin expression by BV associated *Gardnerella vaginalis* and reduces cell cytotoxicity. *Anaerobe*, *50*, 60–63.

Cauci, S. (2004). Vaginal immunity in bacterial vaginosis. *Current Infectious Disease Reports*, 6(6), 450-456.

Cauci, S., & Culhane, J. F. (2007). Modulation of vaginal immune response among pregnant women with bacterial vaginosis by *Trichomonas vaginalis*, *Chlamydia trachomatis*, *Neisseria gonorrhoeae* and yeast. *American Journal of Obstetrics and Gynecolog*, 196(2), 33-1e1 .

Cavicchioli, V. Q., Carvalho, O. V. de, Paiva, J. C. de, Todorov, S. D., Silva Júnior, A., & Nero, L. A. (2018). Inhibition of herpes simplex virus 1 (HSV-1) and poliovirus (PV-1) by bacteriocins from *Lactococcus lactis* subspecies and *Enterococcus durans* strains isolated from goat milk. *International Journal of Antimicrobial Agents*, *51*(1), 33–37.

Cavrois, M., Banerjee, T., Mukherjee, G., Raman, N., Hussien, R., Rodriguez, B. A., … Roan, N. R. (2017). Mass cytometric analysis of HIV entry, replication, and remodeling in tissue CD4+ T Cells. *Cell Reports*, *20*(4), 984–998.

Chang, T. L.-. Y., Chang, C.-. H., Simpson, D. A., Xu, Q., Martin, P. K., Lagenaur, L. A., … Lee, P. P. (2003). Inhibition of HIV infectivity by a natural human isolate of *Lactobacillus jensenii* engineered to express functional two-domain CD4. *Proceedings of the National Academy of Sciences USA*, 100(20), 11672-11677

Cherpes, T. L., Meyn, L. A., Krohn, M. A., Lurie, J. G., & Hillier, S. L. (2003). Association between acquisition of herpes simplex virus type 2 in women and bacterial vaginosis. *Clinical Infectious Diseases*, *37*(3), 319–325.

Chetwin, E., Manhanzva, M. T., Abrahams, A. G., Froissart, R., Gamieldien, H., Jaspan, H., … Masson, L. (2019). Antimicrobial and inflammatory properties of South African clinical *Lactobacillus* isolates and vaginal probiotics. *Scientific Reports*, *9*(1), 1-15.

Cohen, C. R., Lingappa, J. R., Baeten, J. M., Ngayo, M. O., Spiegel, C. A., Hong, T., … Delany, S. (2012). Bacterial vaginosis associated with increased risk of female-to-male HIV-1 transmission: a prospective cohort analysis among African couples. *PLoS Medicine*, 9(6), e1001251.

Cohen, D. P. A., Renes, J., Bouwman, F. G., Zoetendal, E. G., Mariman, E., De Vos, W. M., & Vaughan, E. E. (2006). Proteomic analysis of log to stationary growth phase *Lactobacillus plantarum* cells and a 2-DE database. *Proteomics*, *6*(24), 6485–6493.

Collins, S. L., Mcmillan, A., Seney, S., Veer, C. Van Der, Kort, R., & Sumarah, M. W. (2018). Promising prebiotic candidate established by evaluation of lactitol, lactulose, raffinose, and oligofructose for maintenance of a *Lactobacillus*-dominated vaginal microbiota Stephanie.

Applied and Environmental Microbiology, *84*(5), 1–15.
Cone, R. A. (2008). Barrier properties of mucus. *Advanced Drug Delivery Reviews*, *61*(2), 75–85.
Connor, R. (2006). Sensitivity of non-clade B primary HIV-1 isolates to mildly acidic pH. *Journal of Acquired Immune Deficiency Syndromes*, *43*(4), 499–501.
Conti, C., Malacrino, C., & Mastromarino, P. (2009). Inhibition of herpes simplex virus type 2 by vaginal lactobacilli. *Journal of Physiology and Pharmacology*, *60*(SUPPL.6), 19–26.
Correa, M., & Gisselquist, D. (2006). Routes of HIV transmission in India: assessing the reliability of information from AIDS case surveillance. *International Journal of STD & AIDS*,17(11), 731-735.
Coste, I., Judlin, P., Lepargneur, J.-P., & Bou-Antoun, S. (2012). Safety and efficacy of an intravaginal prebiotic gel in the prevention of recurrent bacterial vaginosis: A randomized double-blind study. *Obstetrics and Gynecology International*, *2012*, 1–7.
Cribby, S., Taylor, M., & Reid, G. (2008). Vaginal microbiota and the use of probiotics. *Interdisciplinary Perspectives on Infectious Diseases*, *2008*, 1–9.
Cu-Uvin, S., Hogan, J. W., Caliendo, A. M., Harwell, J., Mayer, K. H., & Carpenter, C. C. J. (2001). Association between bacterial vaginosis and expression of human immunodeficiency virus type 1 RNA in the female genital tract. *Clinical Infectious Diseases*, 33(6), 894-896.
Damelin, L. H., Paximadis, M., Mavri-Damelin, D., Birkhead, M., Lewis, D. A., & Tiemessen, C. T. (2011). Identification of predominant culturable vaginal *Lactobacillus* species and associated bacteriophages from women with and without vaginal discharge syndrome in South Africa. *Journal of Medical Microbiology*, *60*, 180–183.
Danielsen, M., & Wind, A. (2003). Susceptibility of *Lactobacillus* spp. to antimicrobial agents. *International Journal of Food Microbiology*, *82*(1), 1–11.
Danielsson, D., Teigen, P. K., & Moi, H. (2011). The genital econiche: focus on microbiota and bacterial vaginosis. *Annals of the New York Academy of Sciences*, 1230(1), 48-58.
Danne, C., & Dramsi, S. (2012). Pili of Gram-positive bacteria: Roles in host colonization. *Research in Microbiology*, *163*(9–10), 645–658.
Davar, R., Nokhostin, F., Eftekhar, M., Sekhavat, L., Bashiri Zadeh, M., & Shamsi, F. (2016). Comparing the recurrence of vulvovaginal candidiasis in patients undergoing prophylactic treatment with probiotic and placebo during the 6 Months. *Probiotics and Antimicrobial Proteins*, *8*(3), 130–133.
De Angelis, M., Calasso, M., Cavallo, N., Di Cagno, R., & Gobbetti, M. (2016). Functional proteomics within the genus *Lactobacillus*. *Proteomics*, *16*(6), 946–962.
De Gregorio, P. R., Juárez Tomás, M. S., & Nader-Macías, M. E. F. (2016). Immunomodulation of *Lactobacillus reuteri* CRL1324 on Group B *Streptococcus* vaginal colonization in a murine experimental model. *American Journal of Reproductive Immunology*, *75*(1), 23–35.
de Oliviera, T., Kharshany, A., Graf, T., Cawood, C., Khanyile, D., Grobler, A., … Abdool Karim, S. (2017). Transmission networks and risk of HIV infection in KwaZulu-Natal, South Africa: a community-wide phylogenetic study. *The Lancet HIV*, *4*(1), e41–e50.
Dec, M., Puchalski, A., Urban-Chmiel, R., & Wernicki, A. (2016). 16S-ARDRA and MALDI-TOF mass spectrometry as tools for identification of *Lactobacillus* bacteria isolated from poultry. *Biomed Central Microbiology*, *16*(105).
Dec, M., Urban-Chmiel, R., Gnat, S., Puchalski, A., & Wernicki, A. (2014). Identification of *Lactobacillus* strains of goose origin using MALDI-TOF mass spectrometry and 16S-23S rDNA intergenic spacer PCR analysis. *Research in Microbiology*, *165*(3), 190–201.
Deepika, G., & Charalampopoulos, D. (2010). Surface and adhesion properties of lactobacilli.

Advances in Applied Microbiology, *70*(10), 127–152.

Deese, J., Masson, L., Miller, W., Cohen, M., Morrison, C., Wang, M., … Van Damme, L. (2015). Injectable progestin-only contraception is associated with increased levels of pro-inflammatory cytokines in the female genital tract. *American Journal of Reproductive Immunology*, *74*(4), 357–367.

Dei, M., Di Maggio, F., Di Paolo, G., & Bruni, V. (2010). Vulvovaginitis in childhood. *Best Practice and Research: Clinical Obstetrics and Gynaecology*, *24*(2), 129–137.

Dhanani, A. S., & Bagchi, T. (2013). The roles of moonlighting proteins in bacteria. *Journal of Applied Microbiology*, *115*, 546–554.

Doerflinger, S. Y., Throop, A. L., & Herbst-Kralovetz, M. M. (2014). Bacteria in the vaginal microbiome alter the innate immune response and barrier properties of the human vaginal epithelia in a species-specific manner. *Journal of Infectious Diseases*, *209*(12), 1989–1999.

Drissi, F., Merhej, V., Blanc-Tailleur, C., & Raoult, D. (2015). Draft genome sequence of the *Lactobacillus mucosae* strain Marseille. *Genome Announcements*, *3*(4), 2014–2015. Duskova, M., Ondrej, Š., Zbynek, Z., & Karpískova, R. (2012). Identification of lactobacilli isolated from food by genotypic methods and MALDI-TOF MS. *International Journal of Food Microbiology*, 159(2), 107–114.

Dykes, G. A., & von Holy, A. (1994). Strain typing in the genus *Lactobacillus*. *Letters in Applied Microbiology*, *19*(2), 63–66.

Eastment, M. C., & McClelland, R. S. (2018). Vaginal microbiota and susceptibility to HIV. *Aids*, *32*(6), 687–698.

Eastment, M. C., & R., M. S. (2015). Vaginal microbiota and susceptibility to HIV, *20*(2), 163–178.

Ehrström, S., Daroczy, K., Rylander, E., Samuelsson, C., Johannesson, U., Anzén, B., & Påhlson, C. (2010). Lactic acid bacteria colonization and clinical outcome after probiotic supplementation in conventionally treated bacterial vaginosis and vulvovaginal candidiasis. *Microbes and Infection*, 12(10), 691-699.

El-Adawi, H., Nour, I., Fattouh, F., & El-Deeb, N. (2015). Investigation of the antiviral bioactivity of *Lactobacillus bulgaricus* 761N extracellular extract against hepatitis C virus (HCV). *International Journal of Pharmacology*, *11*(1), 19–26.

Eriksson, K., Carlsson, B., Forsum, U., & Larsson, P. G. (2005). A double-blind treatment study of bacterial vaginosis with normal vaginal lactobacilli after an open treatment with vaginal clindamycin ovules. *Acta Dermato-Venereologica*, *85*(1), 42–46.

Falagas, M. E., Betsi, G. I., & Athanasiou, S. (2007). Probiotics for the treatment of women with bacterial vaginosis. *Clinical Microbiology and Infection*, *13*(7), 657–664.

Fanales-Belasio, E., Raimondo, M., Suligoi, B., & Butto, S. (2010). HIV virology and pathogenetic mechanisms of infection: a brief overview. *Ann Ist Super Sanità*, *46*(1), 5–14.

Fazeli, A., Bruce, C., & Anumba, D. O. (2005). Characterisation of Toll-like receptors in the female reproductive tract in humans. *Human Reproduction*, *20*(5), 1372–1378.

Férir, G., Petrova, M. I., Andrei, G., Huskens, D., Hoorelbeke, B., Snoeck, R., … Schols, D. (2013). The lantibiotic peptide labyrinthopeptin A1 demonstrates broad anti-HIV and Anti-HSV activity with potential for microbicidal applications. *PLoS one*, *8*(5).

Fettweis, J. M., Paul Brooks, J., Serrano, M. G., Sheth, N. U., Girerd, P. H., Edwards, D. J., … Buck, G. A. (2014). Differences in vaginal microbiome in African American women versus women of European ancestry. *Microbiology (United Kingdom)*, *160*(2014), 2272–2282.

Fichorova, R. N., Cronin, A. O., Lien, E., Anderson, D. J., & Ingalls, R. R. (2002). Response to

Neisseria gonorrhoeae by cervicovaginal epithelial cells occurs in the absence of toll-like receptor 4-Mediated Signaling. *The Journal of Immunology*, *168*(5), 2424–2432.

Fichorova, R., Rheinwald, J., & Anderson, D. (1997). Generation of papillomavirus-immortalized cell lines from normal human ectocervical, endocervical, and vaginal epithelium that maintain expression of tissue-specific differentiation proteins. *Biology of Reproduction*, *57*(4), 847–855.

Forsum, U., Hallén, A., & Larsson, P. G. (2005). Bacterial vaginosis - A laboratory and clinical diagnostics enigma: Review article II. *Apmis*, *113*(3), 153–161.

Forsum, U., Holst, E., Larsson, P. G., Vasquez, A., Jakobsson, T., & Mattsbygçébaltzer, I. (2005). Bacterial vaginosis microbiological and immunological enigma. *Apmis*, 113(2), 81-90.

Fredricks, D. N., Fiedler, T. L., & Marrazzo, J. M. (2005). Molecular identification of bacteria associated with bacterial vaginosis. *New England Journal of Medicine*, 353(18), 1899-1911.

Gajer, P., Brotman, R., Bai, G., Sakamoto, J., Schutte, U., Zhong, X., … Ma, Z. (2012). Temporal dynamics of the human vaginal microbiota. *Science Translational Medicine*, *4*(132), 1–21.

Gardiner, G. E., Heinemann, C., Bruce, A. W., Beuerman, D., & Reid, G. (2002). Persistence of *Lactobacillus fermentum* RC-14 and *Lactobacillus rhamnosus* GR-1 but not *L. rhamnosus* GG in the human vagina as demonstrated by randomly amplified polymorphic DNA. *Clinical and Diagnostic Laboratory Immunology*, *9*(1), 92–96.

Gatti, M., Fornasari, E., & Neviani, E. (1997). Cell-wall protein profiles of dairy thermophilic lactobacilli. *Letters in Applied Microbiology*, *25*(5), 345–348.

Gelber, S. E., Aguilar, J. L., Lewis, K. L. T., & Ratner, A. J. (2008). Functional and phylogenetic characterisation of vaginolysin, the human-specific cytolysin from *Gardnerella vaginalis*. *Journal of Bacteriology*, *190*(11), 3896–3903.

Gibson, G. R., & Roberfroid, M. B. (1995). Dietary modulation of the human colonic microbiota: introducing the concept of prebiotics. *The Journal of Nutrition*, *125*(6), 1401–1412.

Gillet, E., Meys, J. F. A., Verstraelen, H., Bosire, C., De Sutter, P., Temmerman, M., & Broeck, D. V. (2011). Bacterial vaginosis is associated with uterine cervical human papillomavirus infection: A meta-analysis. *BMC Infectious Diseases*, 11(10).

Glenting, J., Beck, H. C., Vrang, A., Riemann, H., Ravn, P., Hansen, A. M., … Madsen, S. (2013). Anchorless surface associated glycolytic enzymes from *Lactobacillus plantarum* 299v bind to epithelial cells and extracellular matrix proteins. *Microbiological Research*, 168(5), 245–253.

Goh, Y. J., & Klaenhammer, T. R. (2009). Genomic features of *Lactobacillus* species Yong. *Frontiers in Bioscience*, 14(JAN), 1362–1386.

Gong, Z., Luna, Y., Yu, P., & Fan, H. (2014). Lactobacilli inactivate *Chlamydia trachomatis* through lactic acid but not H_2O_2. *PLoS one*, 9(9), 1–12.

Gosmann, C., Anahtar, M. N., Handley, S. A., Walker, B. D., Virgin, H. W., Kwon, D. S., Bowman, B. A. (2017). *Lactobacillus* -deficient cervicovaginal bacterial communities are associated with increased HIV acquisition in young South African women. *Immunity*, *46*(1), 29–37.

Granato, D., Perotti, F., Masserey, I., Rouvet, M., Golliard, M., Servin, A., & Brassart, D. (1999). Cell surface-associated lipoteichoic acid acts as an adhesion factor for attachment of *Lactobacillus johnsonii* La1 to human enterocyte-like Caco-2 cells. *Applied and Environmental Microbiology*, *65*(3), 1071–1077.

Gueimonde, M., Jalonen, L., He, F., Hiramatsu, M., & Salminen, S. (2006). Adhesion and competitive inhibition and displacement of human enteropathogens by selected lactobacilli. *Food Research International*, 39(4), 467–471.

Gueimonde, M., & Salminen, S. (2006). New methods for selecting and evaluating probiotics. *Digestive and Liver Disease*, *38*(SUPPL. 2), 242–247.

Gupta, K., Scholes, D., & Stamm, W. E. (1999). Increasing prevalence of antimicrobial resistance among uropathogens causing acute uncomplicated cystitis in women. *Acta Veterinaria Scandinavica*, *281*(8), 736–738.

Haggerty, C. L., Hillier, S. L., Bass, D. C., & Ness, R. B. (2004). Bacterial vaginosis and anaerobic bacteria are associated with endometritis. *Clinical Infectious Diseases*, *39*(7), 990–995.

Hanlon, D. E. O., Moench, T. R., Cone, R. A., O'Hanlon, D. E., Moench, T. R., & Cone, R. A. (2011). In vaginal fluid , bacteria associated with bacterial vaginosis can be suppressed with lactic acid but not hydrogen peroxide. *BMC Infectious Diseases*, *11*(1), 200-207.

Happel, A. U., Jaumdally, S. Z., Pidwell, T., Cornelius, T., Jaspan, H. B., Froissart, R., Passmore, J. A. S. (2017). Probiotics for vaginal health in South Africa: What is on retailers' shelves? *BMC Women's Health*, *17*(1), 1–10.

Harrison, A., Colvin, C. J., Kuo, C., Swartz, A., & Lurie, M. (2015). Sustained high HIV incidence in young women in Southern Africa: Social, behavioral, and structural factors and emerging intervention approaches. *Current HIV/AIDS Reports*, *12*(2), 207–215.

Hawes, S. E., Hillier, S. L., Benedetti, J., Stevens, C. E., Koutsky, L. A., Wolner-Hanssen, P., & Holmes, K. K. (1996). Hydrogen peroxide-producing lactobacilli and acquisition of vaginal infections. *Journal of Infectious Diseases*, *174*(5), 1058–1063.

Hay, P. (2009). Recurrent bacterial vaginosis. *Current Opinion in Infectious Diseases*, *22*(1), 82-86.

Hearps, A. C., Tyssen, D., Srbinovski, D., Bayigga, L., Diaz, D. J. D., Aldunate, M., … Tachedjian, G. (2017). Vaginal lactic acid elicits an anti-inflammatory response from human cervicovaginal epithelial cells and inhibits production of pro-inflammatory mediators associated with HIV acquisition. *Mucosal Immunology*, *10*(6), 1480–1490.

Hedge, S. R., Barrientes, F., Desmond, R. A., & Schwebke, J. R. (2006). Local and systemic cytokine levels in relation to changes in vaginal flora. *Journal of Infectious Diseases*, *193*(4), 556-562.

Heinemann, C., & Reid, G. (2005). Vaginal microbial diversity among postmenopausal women with and without hormone replacement therapy. *Canadian Journal of Microbiology*, *51*(9), 777–781.

Heinemann, C., Van Hylckama Vlieg, J. E. T., Janssen, D. B., Busscher, H. J., Van Der Mei, H. C., & Reid, G. (2000). Purification and characterisation of a surface-binding protein from *Lactobacillus fermentum* RC-14 that inhibits adhesion of *Enterococcus faecalis* 1131. *FEMS Microbiology Letters*, *190*(1), 177–180.

Hemalatha, R., Mastromarino, P., Ramalaxmi, B. A., Balakrishna, N. V., & Sesikeran, B. (2012). Effectiveness of vaginal tablets containing lactobacilli versus pH tablets on vaginal health and inflammatory cytokines: A randomized, double-blind study. *European Journal of Clinical Microbiology and Infectious Diseases*, *31*(11), 3097–3105.

Hemmerling, A., Harrison, W., Schroeder, A., Park, J., Korn, A., Shiboski, S., … Cohen, C. R. (2010). Phase 2a study assessing colonization efficiency, safety, and acceptability of *Lactobacillus crispatus* CTV-05 in women with bacterial vaginosis. *Sexually Transmitted Diseases*, *37*(12), 745–750.

Hickey, D. K., Patel, M. V., Fahey, J. V., & Wira, C. R. (2011). Innate and adaptive immunity at mucosal surfaces of the female reproductive tract: Stratification and integration of immune protection against the transmission of sexually transmitted infections. *Journal of Reproductive*

Immunology, *88*(2), 185–194.

Hill, C., Guarner, F., Reid, G., Gibson, G. R., Merenstein, D. J., Pot, B., … Sanders, M. E. (2014). Expert consensus document: The international scientific association for probiotics and prebiotics consensus statement on the scope and appropriate use of the term probiotic. *Nature Reviews Gastroenterology and Hepatology*, *11*(8), 506–514.

Hillier, S. L., Briselden, L. C., & Eschenbach, D. A. (1993). Efficacy of intravaginal 0.75% metronidazole gel for the treatment of bacterial vaginosis. *Obstetrics & Gynecology*, *8*(JUN), *1*(963–967).

Hillier, S. L., Nugent, R. P., Eschenbach, D. A., Krohn, M. A., Gibbs, R. S., Martin, D. H., … Rao, A. V. (1995). Association between bacterial vaginosis and preterm delivery of a low-birth-weight infant. *New England Journal of Medicine*, *333*, 1737-1742

Hladik, F., & Hope, T. J. (2019). HIV infection of the genital mucosa in real time. *Medecine/Sciences*, *6*(1), 20–28.

Hladik, F., Sakchalathorn, P., Ballweber, L., Lentz, G., Fialkow, M., Eschenbach, D., & McElrath, M. J. (2007). Initial events in establishing vaginal entry and infection by human immunodeficiency virus type-1. *Immunity*, *26*(2), 257–270.

Homayouni, A., Bastani, P., Ziyadi, S., Mohammad-Alizadeh-Charandabi, S., Ghalibaf, M., Mortazavian, A. M., & Mehrabany, E. V. (2014). Effects of probiotics on the recurrence of bacterial vaginosis: A review. *Journal of Lower Genital Tract Disease*, *18*(1), 79-86 .

Hu, H., Merenstein, D. J., Wang, C., Hamilton, P. R., Blackmon, M. L., Chen, H., … Li, D. (2013). Impact of eating probiotic yogurt on colonization by candida species of the oral and vaginal mucosa in HIV-infected and HIV-uninfected women. *mycopathologia*, *176*(3–4), 175–181.

Huang, C. H., Chang, M. T., & Huang, L. (2014). Cloning of a novel specific SCAR marker for species identification in *Lactobacillus pentosus*. *Molecular and Cellular Probes*, *28*(4), 192–194.

Hughes, V., & Hillier, S. (1990). Microbiologic characteristics of *Lactobacillus* products used for colonization of the vagina. *Obstetrics and Gynecology*, *75*(2), 244-248.

Hummelen, R., Fernandes, A. D., Macklaim, J. M., Dickson, R. J., Changalucha, J., Gloor, G. B., & Reid, G. (2010). Deep sequencing of the vaginal microbiota of women with HIV. *PLoS one*, *5*(8).

Hütt, P., Shchepetova, J., Lõivukene, K., Kullisaar, T., & Mikelsaar, M. (2006). Antagonistic activity of probiotic lactobacilli and bifidobacteria against entero- and uropathogens. *Journal of Applied Microbiology*, *100*(6), 1324–1332.

Hütt, Pirje, Lapp, E., Štšepetova, J., Smidt, I., Taelma, H., Borovkova, N., … Mändar, R. (2016). Characterisation of probiotic properties in human vaginal lactobacilli strains. *Microbial Ecology in Health & Disease*, *27*(1).

Izquierdo, E., Horvatovich, P., Marchioni, E., Aoude-Werner, D., Sanz, Y., & Ennahar, S. (2009). 2-DE and MS analysis of key proteins in the adhesion of *Lactobacillus plantarum*, a first step toward early selection of probiotics based on bacterial biomarkers. *Electrophoresis*, *30*(6), 949–956.

Janssens, S., & Beyaert, R. (2003). Role of toll-like receptors in pathogen recognition. *Clinical Microbiology Reviews*, *16*(4), 637–646.

Jensen, H., Roos, S., Jonsson, H., Rud, I., Grimmer, S., van Pijkeren, J. P., … Axelsson, L. (2014). Role of *Lactobacillus reuteri* cell and mucus binding protein A (CmbA) in adhesion to intestinal epithelial cells and mucus in vitro. *Microbiology (United Kingdom)*, *160*(PART 4), 671–681.

Jespers, V., Menten, J., Smet, H., Poradosú, S., Abdellati, S., Verhelst, R., … Crucitti, T. (2012). Quantification of bacterial species of the vaginal microbiome in different groups of women , using nucleic acid amplification tests, *12*(83).

Joag, V., Sivro, A., Yende-Zuma, N., Imam, H., Samsunder, N., Karim, Q. A., … Kaul, R. (2018). Ex vivo HIV entry into blood CD4+ T cells does not predict heterosexual HIV acquisition in women. *PLoS one*, *13*(7), 1–12.

Jose, N., Bunt, C., & Hussain, M. (2015). Comparison of microbiological and probiotic characteristics of lactobacilli isolates from dairy food products and animal rumen contents. *Microorganisms*, *3*(2), 198–212.

Jousimies–Somer, H. (1997). Recently described clinically important anaerobic bacteria: Medical aspects. *Clinical Infectious Diseases*, *25*(s2), S88–S93.

Kalichman, S. C., Simbayi, L. C., Kagee, A., Toefy, Y., Jooste, S., Cain, D., & Cherry, C. (2006). Associations of poverty, substance use, and HIV transmission risk behaviors in three South African communities. *Social Science and Medicine*, *62*(7), 1641–1649.

Kankainen, M., Paulin, L., Tynkkynen, S., Von Ossowski, I., Reunanen, J., Partanen, P., … De Vos, W. M. (2009). Comparative genomic analysis of *Lactobacillus rhamnosus* GG reveals pili containing a human-mucus binding protein. *Proceedings of the National Academy of Sciences of the United States of America*, *106*(40), 17193–17198.

Karlsson, M., Scherbak, N., Reid, G., & Jass, J. (2012). *Lactobacillus rhamnosus* GR-1 enhances NF-kappaB activation in *Escherichia coli*-stimulated urinary bladder cells through TLR4. *BMC Microbiology*, *12*(Il), 1–10.

Kaul, R., Nagelkerke, N. J., Kimani, J., Ngugi, E., Bwayo, J. J., MacDonald, K. S., … Moses, S. (2007). Prevalent herpes simplex virus type 2 infection is associated with altered vaginal flora and an increased susceptibility to multiple sexually transmitted infections. *The Journal of Infectious Diseases*, *196*(11), 1692–1697.

Kaushic, C., Ferreira, V. H., Kafka, J. K., & Nazli, A. (2010). HIV infection in the female genital tract: discrete influence of the local mucosal microenvironment. *American Journal of Reproductive Immunology*, *63*(6), 566–575.

Kempf, C., & Jentsch, P. (1991). Inactivation of human immunodeficiency virus (HIV) by low pH and pepsin. *Journal of Acquired Immune Deficiency Syndromes*, *4*(8), 828–830.

Kern, C. C., Vogel, R. F., & Behr, J. (2014). Differentiation of *Lactobacillus brevis* strains using Matrix-Assisted-Laser-Desorption-Ionization-Time-of-flight mass spectrometry with respect to their beer spoilage potential. *Food Microbiology*, *40*(JUN), 18–24.

Kim, Y.-G., Ohta, T., Takahashi, T., Kushiro, A., Nomoto, K., Yokokura, T., … Danbara, H. (2006). Probiotic *Lactobacillus casei* activates innate immunity via NF-κB and p38 MAP kinase signaling pathways. *Microbes and Infection*, *8*(4), 994–1005.

Kirjavainen, P. V., Salminen, S. J., & Isolauri, E. (2003). Probiotic bacteria in the management of atopic disease: Underscoring the importance of viability. *Journal of Pediatric Gastroenterology and Nutrition*, *36*(2), 223–227.

Klatt, N. R., Cheu, R., Birse, K., Zevin, A. S., Perner, M., Noël-romas, L., … Burgener, A. D. (2017b). Vaginal bacteria modify HIV tenofovir microbicide efficacy in African women, *945*(June), 938–945.

Klebanoff, M. A., Schwebke, J. R., Zhang, J., Nansel, T. R., Yu, K. F., & Andrews, W. W. (2004). Vulvovaginal symptoms in women with bacterial vaginosis. *Obstetrics and Gynecology*, *104*(2), 267–272.

Klebanoff, S., Hiller, S., Eschenbach, D., & Waltersdorph, A. (1991). Control of the microbial-flora of the vagina by H_2O_2-generating lactobacilli. *Journal of Infectious Diseases, 164.*

Klebanoff, S. J., & Coombs, R. W. (1991). Viricidal effect of *Lactobacillus acidophilus* on human immunodeficiency virus type 1: possible role in heterosexual transmission. *Journal of Experimental Medicine, 174*(1), 289–292.

Koponen, J., Laakso, K., Koskenniemi, K., Kankainen, M., Savijoki, K., Nyman, T. A., … Varmanen, P. (2012). Effect of acid stress on protein expression and phosphorylation in *Lactobacillus rhamnosus* GG. *Journal of Proteomics, 75*(4), 1357–1374.

Koumans, E H, Sternberg, M., Bruce, C., McQuillan, G., Kendrick, J., Sutton, M., & Markowitz, L. E. (2007). The prevalence of bacterial vaginosis in the United States, 2001-2004; associations with symptoms, sexual behaviors, and reproductive health. *Sexually Transmitted Diseases, 34(11),* 864-869.

Kulakauskas, S., & Marie-Pierre Chapot-Chartier. (2014). Cell wall structure and function in lactic acid bacteria. *Microbial Cell Factories, 13*(Suppl 1), S9.

Kunz, G., Beil, D., Deiniger, H., Einspanier, A., Mall, G., & Leyendecker, G. (1997). Normal and impeded sperm transport within the female genital tract. *The Uterine Peristaltic Pump* (pp. 267–277).

Kwon, D. S., Gregorio, G., Bitton, N., Hendrickson, W. A., & Littman, D. R. (2002). DC-SIGN-mediated internalization of HIV is required for trans-enhancement of T cell infection. *Immunity, 16*(1), 135–144.

Kwong, P. D., Doyle, M. L., Casper, D. J., Cicala, C., Leavitt, S. A., Majeed, S., … Arthos, J. (2002). HIV-1 evades antibody-mediated neutralization through conformational masking of receptor-binding sites. *Nature, 420*(6916), 678–682.

Laakso, K., Koskenniemi, K., Koponen, J., Kankainen, M., Surakka, A., Salusjärvi, T., … Varmanen, P. (2011). Growth phase-associated changes in the proteome and transcriptome of *Lactobacillus rhamnosus* GG in industrial-type whey medium. *Microbial Biotechnology, 4*(6), 746–766.

Lahtinen, S. J., Gueimonde, M., Ouwehand, A. C., Reinikainen, J. P., & Salminen, S. J. (2005). Probiotic bacteria may become dormant during storage. *Applied and Environmental Microbiology, 71*(3), 1662–1663.

Lahtinen, S. J., Gueimonde, M., Ouwehand, A. C., Reinikainen, J. P., & Salminen, S. J. (2006). Comparison of four methods to enumerate probiotic bifidobacteria in a fermented food product. *Food Microbiology, 23*(6), 571–577.

Lai, S. K., Hida, K., Shukair, S., Wang, Y.-Y., Figueiredo, A., Cone, R., … Hanes, J. (2009). Human immunodeficiency virus type 1 is trapped by acidic but not by neutralized human cervicovaginal mucus. *Journal of Virology, 83*(21), 11196–11200.

Larsson, P.-. G., Stray-Pedersen, B., Ryttig, K. R., & Larsen, S. (2008). Human lactobacilli as supplementation of clindamycin to patients with bacterial vaginosis reduce the recurrence rate; a 6-month, double-blind, randomized, placebo-controlled study. *BMC Womens Health, 8*(3), *1-8.*

Larsson, P. G., & Forsum, U. (2005). Bacterial vaginosis - A disturbed bacterial flora and treatment enigma. *Apmis, 113*(5), 305–316.

Lawn, S. D., Butera, S. T., & Folks, T. M. (2001). Contribution of immune activation to the pathogenesis and transmission of human immunodeficiency virus type 1 infection. *Clinical Microbiology Reviews,14*(4), 753–777 .

Lebeer, S., Vanderleyden, J., & De Keersmaecker, S. C. J. (2008). Genes and molecules of lactobacilli supporting probiotic action. *Microbiology and Molecular Biology Reviews, 72*(4),

728–764.

Ledergerber, B., & Battegay, M. (2014). Epidemiology of HIV. *Therapeutische Umschau*, *71*(8), 437–441.

Lederman, M. M., Offord, R. E., & Hartley, O. (2006). Microbicides and other topical strategies to prevent vaginal transmission of HIV. *Nature Reviews Immunology*, *6*, 371–382.

Lee, J., Hwang, K., Jun, W., Park, C., & Lee, M. (2008). Antiinflammatory effect of lactic acid bacteria: inhibition of cyclooxygenase-2 by suppressing nuclear factor-kappaB in Raw264.7 macrophage cells. *Journal of Microbiology and Biotechnology*, *18*(10), 1683–1688.

Lennard, K., Dabee, S., Barnabas, S. L., Havyarimana, E., Blakney, A., Jaumdally, S. Z., … Jaspana, H. B. (2018). Microbial composition predicts genital tract inflammation and persistent bacterial vaginosis in South African adolescent females. *Infection and Immunity*, *86*(1).

Ling, Z., Liu, X., Chen, W., Luo, Y., Yuan, L., Xia, Y., … Xiang, C. (2013). The restoration of the vaginal microbiota after treatment for bacterial vaginosis with metronidazole or probiotics. *Microbial Ecology*, *65*(3), 773–780.

Lorca, G., Torino, M. I., Font De Valdez, G., & Ljungh, Å. (2002). Lactobacilli express cell surface proteins which mediate binding of immobilized collagen and fibronectin. *FEMS Microbiology Letters*, *206*(1), 31–37.

Luster, A. D. (2002). The role of chemokines in linking innate and adaptive immunity. *Current Opinion in Immunology*, *14*(1), 129–135.

Machado, D., Castro, J., Palmeira-de-Oliveira, A., Martinez-de-Oliveira, J., & Cerca, N. (2016). Bacterial vaginosis biofilms: Challenges to current therapies and emerging solutions. *Frontiers in Microbiology*, *6*(1528).

MacKenzie, D. A., Jeffers, F., Parker, M. L., Vibert-Vallet, A., Bongaerts, R. J., Roos, S., … Juge, N. (2010). Strain-specific diversity of mucus-binding proteins in the adhesion and aggregation properties of *Lactobacillus reuteri*. *Microbiology*, *156*(11), 3368–3378.

Macklaim, J. M., Clemente, J. C., Knight, R., Gloor, G. B., & Reid, G. (2015). Changes in vaginal microbiota following antimicrobial and probiotic therapy. *Microbial Ecology in Health & Disease*, *26*(0).

Macklaim, J. M., Gloor, G. B., Anukam, K. C., Cribby, S., & Reid, G. (2011). At the crossroads of vaginal health and disease, the genome sequence of *Lactobacillus iners* AB-1. *Proceedings of the National Academy of Sciences of the United States of America*, *108*(SUPPL. 1), 4688–4695.

Maher, D., Wu, X., Schacker, T., Horbul, J., & Southern, P. (2005). HIV binding, penetration, and primary infection in human cervicovaginal tissue. *Proceedings of the National Academy of Sciences of the United States of America*, *102*(32), 11504–11509.

Marco, M. L., Pavan, S., & Kleerebezem, M. (2006). Towards understanding molecular modes of probiotic action. *Current Opinion in Biotechnology*, *17*(2), 204–210.

Marcone, V., Calzolari, E., & Bertini, M. (2008). Effectiveness of vaginal administration of *Lactobacillus rhamnosus* following conventional metronidazole therapy: How to lower the rate of bacterial vaginosis recurrences. *New Microbiologica*, *31*(3), 429–433.

Marks, G., Gardner, L. I., Rose, C. E., Zinski, A., Moore, R. D., Rodriguez, A. E., … Affairs, V. (2016). Time above 1500 copies: a viral load measure for assessing transmission risk of HIV-positive patients in care, *29*(8), 947–954.

Marrazzo, J. M., Ramjee, G., Richardson, B. A., Gomez, K., Mgodi, N., Nair, G., … Chirenje, Z. M. (2015). Tenofovir-based preexposure prophylaxis for HIV infection among African women. *New England Journal of Medicine*, *372*(6), 509–518.

Martin, R., & Suírez, J. E. (2010). Biosynthesis and degradation of H2O2 by vaginal lactobacilli. *Applied and Environmental Microbiology, 76*(2), 400-405.

Martin, L. S., McDougal, S. J., & Loskoski, S. L. (1985). Disinfection and inactivation of the human T lymphotropic virus type III / lymphadenopathy-associated virus. *The Journal of Infectious Diseases*, *152*(2), 400–403.

Martínez-Peña, M. D., Castro-Escarpulli, G., & Aguilera-Arreola, M. G. (2013). *Lactobacillus* species isolated from vaginal secretions of healthy and bacterial vaginosis-intermediate Mexican women: A prospective study. *BMC Infectious Diseases*, *13*(189).

Masson, L., Arnold, K. B., Little, F., Mlisana, K., Lewis, D. A., Mkhize, N., … Passmore, J.-A. S. (2016). Inflammatory cytokine biomarkers to identify women with asymptomatic sexually transmitted infections and bacterial vaginosis who are at high risk of HIV infection. *Sexually Transmitted Infections*, *92*(3), 186–193.

Masson, L., Mlisana, K., Little, F., Werner, L., Mkhize, N. N., Ronacher, K., … Walzl, G. (2014). Defining genital tract cytokine signatures of sexually transmitted infections and bacterial vaginosis in women at high risk of HIV infection: a cross-sectional study. *Sexually Transmitted Infections, 90*(8) 580-587.

Masson, L., Passmore, J.-A. S., Liebenberg, L. J., Werner, L., Baxter, C., Arnold, K. B., … Abdool Karim, S. S. (2015). Genital inflammation and the risk of HIV acquisition in women. *Clinical Infectious Diseases*, *61*(2), 260–269.

Mastromarino, P, Brigidi, P., Macchia, S., Maggi, L., & Pirovano, F. (2002). Characterisation and selection of vaginal *Lactobacillus* strains for the preparation of vaginal tablets, 884–893.

Mastromarino, Paola, Cacciotti, F., Masci, A., & Mosca, L. (2011). Antiviral activity of *Lactobacillus brevis* towards herpes simplex virus type 2: Role of cell wall associated components. *Anaerobe*, *17*(6), 334–336.

Mastromarino, Paola, Macchia, S., Meggiorini, L., Trinchieri, V., Mosca, L., Perluigi, M., & Midulla, C. (2009). Effectiveness of *Lactobacillus*-containing vaginal tablets in the treatment of symptomatic bacterial vaginosis. *Clinical Microbiology and Infection*, *15*(1), 67–74.

Mastromarino, Paola, Vitali, B., & Mosca, L. (2013). Bacterial vaginosis: a review on clinical trials with probiotics. *The New Microbiologica*, *36*, 229–238.

Mayer-Barber, K. D., & Yan, B. (2017). Clash of the Cytokine Titans: Counter-regulation of interleukin-1 and type i interferon-mediated inflammatory responses. *Cellular and Molecular Immunology*, *14*(1), 22–35.

McClelland, R. S., Lingappa, J. R., Srinivasan, S., Kinuthia, J., John-Stewart, G. C., Jaoko, W., … Fredricks, D. N. (2018). Evaluation of the association between the concentrations of key vaginal bacteria and the increased risk of HIV acquisition in African women from five cohorts: a nested case-control study. *The Lancet Infectious Diseases*, *18*(5), 554–564.

Mcinnes, I. B. Cytokines, Chapter 26, p396.

McKinnon, L. R., Achilles, S. L., Bradshaw, C. S., Burgener, A., Crucitti, T., Fredricks, D. N., … Tachedjian, G. (2019). The evolving facets of bacterial vaginosis: Implications for HIV transmission. *AIDS Research and Human Retroviruses*, *35*(3), 219–228.

McKinnon, L. R., Liebenberg, L. J., Yende-Zuma, N., Archary, D., Ngcapu, S., Sivro, A., … Passmore, J. A. S. (2018). Genital inflammation undermines the effectiveness of tenofovir gel in preventing HIV acquisition in women. *Nature Medicine*, *24*(4), 491–496.

Mclean I.J., N. W. . R. (2000). Characterisation and selection of a *Lactobacillus* species to re-colonize the vagina of women with recurrent bacterial vaginosis. *Journal of Medical*

Microbiology, *49*(2000), 543–552.

Mclean, N. W., & Mcgroarty, J. A. (1996). Growth inhibition of metronidazole-susceptible and metronidazole-resistant strains of *Gardnerella vaginalis* by lactobacilli in vitro. *Applied and Environmental Microbiology*, *62*(3), 1089–1092.

McLean, N. W., & Rosenstein, I. J. (2000). Characterisation and selection of a *Lactobacillus* species to re-colonise the vagina of women with recurrent bacterial vaginosis. *Journal of Medical Microbiology*, *49*(6), 543-552 .

Miller, C. J., Li, Q., Abel, K., Kim, E.-Y., Ma, Z.-M., Wietgrefe, S., … Haase, A. T. (2005). Propagation and dissemination of infection after vaginal transmission of simian immunodeficiency virus. *Journal of Virology*, *79*(17), 11552–11552.

Mirmonsef, P., Gilbert, D., Zariffard, M. R., Hamaker, B. R., Kaur, A., Landay, A. L., & Spear, G. T. (2011). The effects of commensal bacteria on innate immune responses in the female genital tract. *American Journal of Reproductive Immunology*, *65*(3), 190–195.

Mirmonsef, P., Modur, S., Burgad, D., Gilbert, D., Golub, E. T., French, A. L., … Alan, L. (2016). An exploratory comparison of vaginal glycogen and *Lactobacillus* level in pre- and post-menopouse women. *Menopouse*, *22*(7), 702–709.

Miyoshi, Y., Okada, S., Uchimura, T., & Satoh, E. (2006). A mucus adhesion promoting protein, MapA, mediates the adhesion of *Lactobacillus reuteri* to Caco-2 human intestinal epithelial cells. *Bioscience, Biotechnology and Biochemistry*, *70*(7), 1622–1628.

Mlisana, K., Naicker, N., Werner, L., Roberts, L., Van Loggerenberg, F., Baxter, C., … Abdool Karim, S. S. (2012). Symptomatic vaginal discharge is a poor predictor of sexually transmitted infections and genital tract inflammation in high-risk women in South Africa. *Journal of Infectious Diseases*, *206*(1), 6–14.

Mohanty, S., Sood, S., Kapil, A., & Mittal, S. (2010). Interobserver variation in the interpretation of Nugent scoring method for diagnosis of bacterial vaginosis. *Indian Journal of Medical Research*, *131*(1), 88–91.

Moore, J. P. (1997). Coreceptors-Implications for HIV pathogenesis and therapy. *Science*, *276*(5309), 51 LP – 52.

Morrison, C., Fichorova, R. N., Mauck, C., Chen, P. L., Kwok, C., Chipato, T., … Doncel, G. F. (2014). Cervical inflammation and immunity associated with hormonal contraception, pregnancy, and HIV-1 seroconversion. *Journal of Acquired Immune Deficiency Syndromes*, *66*(2), 109–117.

Muzio, M., Natoli, G., Saccani, S., Levrero, M., & Mantovani, A. (1998). The human toll signaling pathway: Divergence of nuclear factor κb and jnk/sapk activation upstream of tumor necrosis factor receptor-associated factor 6 (TRAF6). *Journal of Experimental Medicine*, *187*(12), 2097–2101.

ñahui Palomino, R. A., Zicari, S., Vanpouille, C., Vitali, B., & Margolis, L. (2017). Vaginal *Lactobacillus* inhibits HIV-1 replication in human tissues ex vivo. *Frontiers in Microbiology*, *8*(MAY), 1–11.

Nardini, P., Ñãhui Palomino, R. A., Parolin, C., Laghi, L., Foschi, C., Cevenini, R., … Marangoni, A. (2016). *Lactobacillus crispatus* inhibits the infectivity of *Chlamydia trachomatis* elementary bodies, in vitro study. *Scientific Reports*, *6*(February), 1–11.

Nasioudis, D., Linhares, I. M., Ledger, W. J., & Witkin, S. S. (2016). Bacterial vaginosis: a critical analysis of current knowledge. *BJOG: An International Journal of Obstetrics and Gynaecology*, *124*(1), 61–69.

Nasioudis, D., Linhares, I. M., Ledger, W. J., & Witkin, S. S. (2017). Bacterial vaginosis: a critical analysis of current knowledge. *BJOG: An International Journal of Obstetrics and Gynaecology*, *124*(1), 61–69.

Nasu, K., & Narahara, H. (2010). Pattern recognition via the toll-like receptor system in the human female genital tract. *Mediators of Inflammation, 2010(*976024).

Nazli, A., Chan, O., Dobson-Belaire, W. N., Ouellet, M., Tremblay, M. J., Gray-Owen, S. D., … Kaushic, C. (2010). Exposure to HIV-1 directly impairs mucosal epithelial barrier integrity allowing microbial translocation. *PLoS Pathogens*, *6*(4), e1000852.

Ness, R. B., Kip, K. E., Hillier, S. L., Soper, D. E., Stamm, C. A., Sweet, R. L., … Richter, H. E. (2005). A cluster analysis of bacterial vaginosis-associated microflora and pelvic inflammatory disease. *American Journal of Epidemiology*, *162*(6), 585–590.

Nishiyama, K., Nakazato, A., Ueno, S., Seto, Y., Kakuda, T., Takai, S., … Mukai, T. (2015). Cell surface-associated aggregation-promoting factor from *Lactobacillus gasseri*SBT2055 facilitates host colonization and competitive exclusion of *Campylobacter jejuni*. *Molecular Microbiology*, *98*(4), 712–726.

Nugent, R. P., Krohn, M. A., & Hillier, S. L. (1991). Reliability of diagnosing bacterial vaginosis is improved by a standardized method of gram stain interpretation. *Journal of Clinical Microbiology*, *29*(2), 97-301.

Nunn, K. L., & Forney, L. J. (2016). Unraveling the dynamics of the human vaginal microbiome. *Yale Journal of Biology and Medicine*, *89*(3), 331–337.

Nygaard, V., Rødland, E. A., & Hovig, E. (2016). Methods that remove batch effects while retaining group differences may lead to exaggerated confidence in downstream analyses. *Biostatistics*, *17*(1), 29–39.

O'Connor, T. J., Kinchington, D., Kangro, H. O., & Jeffries, D. J. (1995). The activity of candidate virucidal agents, low pH and genital secretions against HIV-1 in vitro. *International Journal of STD & AIDS*, *6*(4).

O'Hanlon, D E, Moench, T. R., & Cone, R. A. (2011). In vaginal fluid, bacteria associated with bacterial vaginosis can be suppressed with lactic acid but not hydrogen peroxide. *BMC Infectious Diseases*, *11*(1), 200–207.

O'Hanlon, D. E., Lanier, B. R., Moench, T. R., & Cone, R. A. (2010). Cervicovaginal fluid and semen block the microbicidal activity of hydrogen peroxide produced by vaginal lactobacilli. *BMC Infectious Diseases*, *10*(120).

O'Hanlon, D. E., Moench, T. R., & Cone, R. A. (2013). Vaginal pH and microbicidal lactic acid when lactobacilli dominate the microbiota. *PLoS one*, *8*(11), 1–8.

Ocana, V. S. (1999). Selection of vaginal H_2O_2 -generating *Lactobacillus* species for probiotic use, *38*, 279–284.

Onywera, H., Williamson, A. L., Mbulawa, Z. Z. A., Coetzee, D., & Meiring, T. L. (2019). The cervical microbiota in reproductive-age South African women with and without human papillomavirus infection. *Papillomavirus Research*, *7*(December 2018), 154–163.

Osborn, L., Kunkel, S., & Nabel, G. J. (1989a). Tumor necrosis factor-α and interleukin-1 stimulate the human immunodeficiency virus enhancer by activation of the nuclear factor κ B. *Proceedings of the National Academy of Sciences*, *86*(7), 2336–2340.

Osset, J., Bartolomé, R. M., García, E., & Andreu, A. (2001). Assessment of the capacity of *Lactobacillus* to inhibit the growth of uropathogens and block their adhesion to vaginal epithelial cells. *The Journal of Infectious Diseases*, *183*(3), 485–491.

Özcelik, S., Kuley, E., & Özogul, F. (2016). Formation of lactic, acetic, succinic, propionic, formic and butyric acid by lactic acid bacteria. *LWT - Food Science and Technology*, *73*, 536–542.

Patterson, J. L., Stull-Lane, A., Girerd, P. H., & Jefferson, K. K. (2010). Analysis of adherence, biofilm formation and cytotoxicity suggests a greater virulence potential of *Gardnerella vaginalis* relative to other bacterial-vaginosis-associated anaerobes. *Microbiology*, *156*(2), 392–399.

Pavlova, S. I., Kilic, A. O., Kilic, S. S., So, J. S., Nader-Macias, M. E., Simoes, J. A., & Tao, L. (2002). Genetic diversity of vaginal lactobacilli from women in different countries based on 16S rRNA gene sequences. *Journal of Applied Microbiology*, *92*(3), 451–459.

Pendharkar, S., Magopane, T., Larsson, P.-G., Bruyn, G. de, Gray, G. E., Hammarström, L., & Marcotte, H. (2013a). Identification and characterisation of vaginal lactobacilli from South African women. *BMC Infectious Diseases*, *13*(1), 43.

Pendharkar, S., Magopane, T., Larsson, P.-G., Bruyn, G. de, Gray, G. E., Hammarström, L., & Marcotte, H. (2013b). Identification and characterisation of vaginal lactobacilli from South African women. *BMC Infectious Diseases*, *13*(1), 43.

Pérez Montoro, B., Benomar, N., Caballero Gómez, N., Ennahar, S., Horvatovich, P., Knapp, C. W., … Abriouel, H. (2018). Proteomic analysis of *Lactobacillus pentosus* for the identification of potential markers of adhesion and other probiotic features. *Food Research International*, *111*(April), 58–66.

Petricevic, L., & Witt, A. (2008). The role of *Lactobacillus casei rhamnosus* Lcr35 in restoring the normal vaginal flora after antibiotic treatment of bacterial vaginosis. *BJOG: An International Journal of Obstetrics and Gynaecology*, *115*(11), 1369–1374.

Petrova, M. I., Lievens, E., Malik, S., Imholz, N., & Lebeer, S. (2015). *Lactobacillus* species as biomarkers and agents that can promote various aspects of vaginal health. *Frontiers in Physiology*, *6*(MAR), 1–18.

Petrova, M. I., Reid, G., Vaneechoutte, M., & Lebeer, S. (2017). *Lactobacillus iners*: Friend or foe? *Trends in Microbiology*, *25*(3), 182–191.

Petrova, M. I., van den Broek, M., Balzarini, J., Vanderleyden, J., & Lebeer, S. (2013). Vaginal microbiota and its role in HIV transmission and infection. *FEMS Microbiology Reviews*, *37*(5), 762-792.

Pino, A., Bartolo, E., Caggia, C., Cianci, A., & Randazzo, C. L. (2019). Detection of vaginal lactobacilli as probiotic candidates. *Scientific Reports*, *9*(1), 1–10.

Pope, M., & Haase, A. T. (2003). Transmission, acute HIV-1 infection and the quest for strategies to prevent infection. *Nature Medicine*, *9*, 847–852.

Thomas C. Q., Maria J. W., Nelson S., *et al* (2000). Viral load and heterosexual transmission of human immuno deficiency virus type 1, *342*(13) 921–929.

Pot, B., Hertel, C., Ludwig, W., & Descheemaeker, P. (1993). Identification and classification of *Lactobacillus acidophilus*, *L. gasseri* and *L. johnsonii* strains by SDS-PAGE and rRNA-targeted oligonucleotide probe hybridization. *Journal of General Microbiology*, (1993), 5–9.

Powers, K. A., Poole, C., Pettifor, A. E., & Cohen, M. S. (2008). Rethinking the heterosexual infectivity of HIV-1: a systematic review and meta-analysis. *The Lancet Infectious Diseases*, *8*(9), 553–563.

Pudney, J., Quayle, A. J., & Anderson, D. J. (2005). Immunological microenvironments in the human vagina and cervix: mediators of cellular immunity are concentrated in the cervical transformation zone1. *Biology of Reproduction*, *73*(6), 1253–1263.

Quayle, A. J. (2002). The innate and early immune response to pathogen challenge in the female genital tract and the pivotal role of epithelial cells. *Journal of Reproductive Immunology*, *57*(1–2), 61–79.

Qureshi, T. A., Mirbahar, K. B., Samo, M. U., Soomro, N. M., Solangi, A. A., & Memon, A. (2006). Clinical study of experimentally induced anaphylactic shock in goats. *International Journal of Pharmacology*, *2*(3), 357–361.

Ramiah, K., van Reenen, C. A., & Dicks, L. M. T. (2008). Surface-bound proteins of *Lactobacillus plantarum* 423 that contribute to adhesion of Caco-2 cells and their role in competitive exclusion and displacement of *Clostridium sporogenes* and *Enterococcus faecalis*. *Research in Microbiology*, *159*(6), 470–475.

Randelović, G., Mladenović, V., Ristić, L., Otašević, S., Branković, S., Mladenović-Antić, S., … Bogdanović, D. (2012). Microbiological aspects of vulvovaginitis in prepubertal girls. *European Journal of Pediatrics*, *171*(8), 1203–1208.

Rapisarda, A. M. C., Caldaci, L., Valenti, G., Brescia, R., Sapia, F., Sarpietro, G., … Panella, M. M. (2018). Efficacy of vaginal preparation containing *Lactobacillus acidophilus*, lactic acid and deodorized garlic extract in treatment and prevention of symptomatic bacterial vaginitis: Result from a single-arm pilot study. *Italian Journal of Gynaecology and Obstetrics*, *30*(1), 21–31.

Rathod, S. D., Krupp, K., Klausner, J. D., Arun, A., Reingold, A. L., & Madhivanan, P. (2012). Bacterial vaginosis and risk for *Trichomonas vaginalis* infection. *Sexually Transmitted Diseases*, *39*(6), 493.

Ravel, J., Gajer, P., Abdo, Z., Schneider, G. M. M., Koenig, S. S. K., McCulle, S. L., … Forney, L. J. (2011). Vaginal microbiome of reproductive-age women. *Proceedings of the National Academy of Sciences*, *108*(Supplement 1), 4680–4687.

Ravula, R. R., & Shah, N. P. (1998). Effect of acid casein hydrolysate and cysteine on the viability of ... *Australian Journal of Dairy Technology*, *53*(3), 175.

Raz, R., Colodner, R., Rohana, Y., Battino, S., Rottensterich, E., Wasser, I., & Stamm, W. (2003). Effectiveness of estriol-containing vaginal pessaries and nitrofurantoin macrocrystal therapy in the prevention of recurrent urinary tract infection in postmenopausal women. *Clinical Infectious Diseases*, *36*(11), 1362–1368.

Reid, G., Beuerman, D., Heinemann, C., & Bruce, A. W. (2001). Probiotic *Lactobacillus* dose required to restore and maintain a normal vaginal flora. *FEMS Immunology & Medical Microbiology*, *32*(1), 37-41.

Reid, G., Jass, J., Sebulsky, M. T., & Mccormick, J. K. (2003). Potential uses of probiotics in clinical practice. *Clinical Microbiology Reviews*, *16*(4), 658–672.

Rivas-Sendra, A., Landete, J. M., Alcántara, C., & Zúñiga, M. (2011). Response of *Lactobacillus casei* BL23 to phenolic compounds. *Journal of Applied Microbiology*, *111*(6), 1473–1481.

Rizzuto, C. D., & Sodroski, J. G. (1997). Contribution of virion ICAM-1 to human immunodeficiency virus infectivity and sensitivity to neutralization. *Journal of Virology*, *71*(6), 4847–4851.

Robboy, S. J., & Bentley, R. C. (2004). *Histology for pathologists*. 2nd edition

Rose, W. A., McGowin, C. L., Spagnuolo, R. A., Eaves-Pyles, T. D., Popov, V. L., & Pyles, R. B. (2012). Commensal bacteria modulate innate immune responses of vaginal epithelial cell multilayer cultures. *PLoS one*, *7*(3).

Rousseau, V., Lepargneur, J. P., Roques, C., Remaud-Simeon, M., & Paul, F. (2005). Prebiotic effects of oligosaccharides on selected vaginal lactobacilli and pathogenic microorganisms. *Anaerobe*, *11*(3), 145–153.

Ryckman, K. K., Williams, S. M., Krohn, M. A., & Simhan, H. N. (2008). Racial differences in cervical cytokine concentrations between pregnant women with and without bacterial vaginosis. *Journal of Reproductive Immunology*, *78*(2), 166–171.

Saad, N., Urdaci, M., Vignoles, C., Chaignepain, S., Tallon, R., Schmitter, J. M., & Bressollier, P. (2009). *Lactobacillus plantarum* 299v surface-bound GAPDH: A new insight into enzyme cell walls location. *Journal of Microbiology and Biotechnology*, *19*(12), 1635–1643.

Saeed, S., Rasool, S. A., Ahmad, S., Zaid, S. Z., & Rehmani, S. (2007). Antiviral activity of Staphylococcin 188: A purified bacteriocin like inhibitory substance isolated from *Staphylococcus aureus* AB188, *Research Journal of Microbiology* *2*(11), 796-806.

Samuel, K., Taelma, H., Štšepetova, J., Borovkova, N., Hoidmets, D., Lapp, E., … Salumets, A. (2016). Characterisation of probiotic properties in human vaginal lactobacilli strains. *Microbial Ecology in Health and Disease*, *27*(30484).

Sanders, M. E. (2008). Probiotics: Definition, Sources, Selection, and Uses. *Clinical Infectious Diseases*, *46*(s2), S58–S61.

Santarmaki, V., Kourkoutas, Y., Zoumpopoulou, G., Mavrogonatou, E., Kiourtzidis, M., Chorianopoulos, N., … Ypsilantis, P. (2017). Survival, intestinal mucosa adhesion, and immunomodulatory potential of *Lactobacillus plantarum* strains. *Current Microbiology*, *74*(9), 1061–1067.

Santos, C. M. A., Pires, M. C. V., Leão, T. L., Silva, A. K. S., Miranda, L. S., Martins, F. S., … Nicoli, J. R. (2018). Anti-inflammatory effect of two *Lactobacillus* strains during infection with *Gardnerella vaginalis* and *Candida albicans* in a hela cell culture model. *Microbiology (United Kingdom)*, *164*(3), 349–358.

Sarafianos, S. G., Marchand, B., Das, K., Himmel, D. M., Parniak, M. A., Hughes, S. H., & Arnold, E. (2009). Structure and function of HIV-1 reverse transcriptase: Molecular mechanisms of polymerization and inhibition. *Journal of Molecular Biology*, *385*(3), 693–713.

Sato, H., Torimura, M., Kitahara, M., Ohkuma, M., Hotta, Y., & Tamura, H. (2012). Characterisation of the *Lactobacillus casei* group based on the profiling of ribosomal proteins coded in S10-spc-alpha operons as observed by MALDI-TOF MS. *Systematic and Applied Microbiology*, *35*(7), 447–454.

Schwebke, J. R. (2009). New concepts in the etiology of bacterial vaginosis. *Current Infectious Disease Reports*, *11*(2), 143–147.

Schwebke, J. R., Gaydos, C. A., Nyirjesy, P., Paradis, S., Kodsi, S., & Cooper, C. K. (2018). Diagnostic performance of a molecular test versus clinician assessment of vaginitis. *Journal of Clinical Microbiology*, *56*(6), 1–13.

Serkedjieva, J., Danova, S., & Ivanova, I. (2000). Antiinfluenza virus activity of a bacteriocin produced by *Lactobacillus delbrueckii*. *Applied Biochemistry and Biotechnology - Part A Enzyme Engineering and Biotechnology*, *88*(1–3), 285–298.

Sgibnev, V., & Kremleva, A. (2015). Vaginal protection by hydrogen peroxide-producing lactobacilli. *Jundishapur Journal of Microbiology*, *8*(10), e22913

De Man J. C., Rogosa M., Sharpe M.E., (1960). A medium for the cultivation of lactobacilli. *Applied Microbiology*, *23*(1), 130–135.

Shaw, G. M., & Hunter, E. (2012). HIV Transmission. *Cold Spring Harbor Perspectives in Medicine*.

Shenoy, A., & Gottlieb, A. (2019). Probiotics for oral and vulvovaginal candidiasis: A Review. *Dermatologic Therapy*, *32*(4) e12970.

Shi, Y., Chen, L., Tong, J., & Xu, C. (2009). Preliminary characterisation of vaginal microbiota in healthy Chinese women using cultivation-independent methods. *Journal of Obstetrics and Gynaecology Research*, *35*(3), 525–532.

Simon, V., Ho, D. D., & Karim, Q. A. (2006). HIV/AIDS epidemiology, pathogenesis, prevention, and treatment. *The Lancet, 368*(9534), 489-504.

Siragusa, S., De Angelis, M., Calasso, M., Campanella, D., Minervini, F., Di Cagno, R., & Gobbetti, M. (2014). Fermentation and proteome profiles of *Lactobacillus plantarum* strains during growth under food-like conditions. *Journal of Proteomics*, *96*, 366–380.

Srinivasan, S., & Fredricks, D. N. (2008). The human vaginal bacterial biota and bacterial vaginosis. *Interdisciplinary Perspectives on Infectious Diseases*, *2008*, 1–22.

Srinivasan, S., Hoffman, N. G., Morgan, M. T., Matsen, F. A., Fiedler, T. L., Hall, R. W., … Fredricks, D. N. (2012). Bacterial communities in women with bacterial vaginosis: high resolution phylogenetic analyses reveal relationships of microbiota to clinical criteria. *PLoS one*, *7*(6), e37818.

St. John, E. P., Martinson, J., Simoes, J. A., Landay, A. L., & Spear, G. T. (2007). Dendritic cell activation and maturation induced by mucosal fluid from women with bacterial vaginosis. *Clinical Immunology*, *125*(1), 95–102.

Stamey, T. A., & Timothy, M. M. (1975). Studies of introital colonization in women with recurrent urinary infections. I. The role of vaginal pH. *Journal of Urology*, *114*(2), 261–263.

Stoddard, E., Ni, H., Cannon, G., Zhou, C., Kallenbach, N., Malamud, D., & Weissman, D. (2010). Gp340 promotes transcytosis of human immunodeficiency virus type 1 in genital tract-derived cell lines and primary endocervical tissue. *Journal of Viral Entry*, *4*(1), 27–28.

Strömbeck, L., Sandros, J., Holst, E., Madianos, P., Nannmark, U., Papapanou, P., & Mattsby-Baltzer, I. (2007). *Prevotella bivia* can invade human cervix epithelial (HeLa) cells. *Apmis*, *115*(3), 241–251.

Sutherland, A., Tester, R., Al-Ghazzewi, F., McCulloch, E., & Connolly, M. (2008). Glucomannan hydrolysate (GMH) inhibition of *Candida albicans* growth in the presence of *Lactobacillus* and *Lactococcus* species. *Microbial Ecology in Health and Disease*, *20*(3), 127–134.

Svanborg, C., Godaly, G., & Hedlund, M. (1999). Cytokine responses during mucosal infections: Role in disease pathogenesis and host defence. *Current Opinion in Microbiology*, *2*(1), 99–103.

Tachedjian, G., Aldunate, M., Bradshaw, C. S., & Cone, R. A. (2017). The role of lactic acid production by probiotic *Lactobacillus* species in vaginal health. *Research in Microbiology*, *168*(9–10), 782–792.

Taha, T E, Hoover, D. R., Dallabetta, G. A., Kumwenda, N. I., Mtimavalye, L. A., Yang, L. P., … Miotti, P. G. (1998). Bacterial vaginosis and disturbances of vaginal biota: association with increased acquisition of HIV. *AIDS*, *12*(13), *1699-1706*. .

Takebe, Y. (2001). HIV-1 Genetic diversity : Mechanism and its biological implication. *Uirusu*, *51*(2), 123–134.

Tamrakar, R., Yamada, T., Furuta, I., Cho, K., Morikawa, M., Yamada, H., … Minakami, H. (2007). Association between *Lactobacillus* species and bacterial vaginosis-related bacteria, and bacterial vaginosis scores in pregnant Japanese women. *BMC Infectious Diseases*, *7*(128).

Tang, D., Kang, R., Coyne, C. B., Zeh, H. J., & Lotze, M. T. (2012). PAMPs and DAMPs: Signal 0s that spur autophagy and immunity. *Immunological Reviews*, *249*(1), 158–175.

Tärnberg, M., Jakobsson, T., Jonasson, J., & Forsum, U. (2002). Identification of randomly selected colonies of lactobacilli from normal vaginal fluid by pyrosequencing of the 16S rDNA variable V1 and V3 regions. *Apmis*, *110*(11), 802–810.

Taweechotipatr, M., Iyer, C., Spinler, J. K., Versalovic, J., & Tumwasorn, S. (2009). *Lactobacillus saerimneri* and *Lactobacillus ruminis*: Novel human-derived probiotic strains with immunomodulatory activities. *FEMS Microbiology Letters*, *293*(1), 65–72.

Temmerman, R., Pot, B., Huys, G., & Swings, J. (2003). Identification and antibiotic susceptibility of bacterial isolates from probiotic products available in Italy. *International Journal of Food Microbiology*, *81*(4), 1–10.

Thies, F. L., König, W., & König, B. (2007). Rapid characterisation of the normal and disturbed vaginal microbiota by application of 16S rRNA gene terminal RFLP fingerprinting. *Journal of Medical Microbiology*, *56*(6), 755–761.

Thurman, A. R., & Doncel, G. F. (2011). Innate immunity and inflammatory response to *Trichomonas vaginalis* and bacterial vaginosis: Relationship to HIV acquisition. *American Journal of Reproductive Immunology*, *65*(2), 89–98.

Tobita, K., Watanabe, I., & Saito, M. (2016). Specific vaginal lactobacilli suppress the inflammation induced by lipopolysaccharide stimulation through downregulation of toll-like receptor expression in human embryonic intestinal epithelial cells. *Bioscience of Microbiota, Food and Health*, *36*(1), 39–44.

Todorov, Svetoslav D., Wachsman, M. B., Knoetze, H., Meincken, M., & Dicks, L. M. T. (2005). An antibacterial and antiviral peptide produced by *Enterococcus mundtii* ST4V isolated from soya beans. *International Journal of Antimicrobial Agents*, *25*(6), 508–513.

Todorov, Svetoslav Dimitrov, Wachsman, M., Tomé, E., Dousset, X., Destro, M. T., Dicks, L. M. T., … Drider, D. (2010). Characterisation of an antiviral pediocin-like bacteriocin produced by *Enterococcus faecium*. *Food Microbiology*, *27*(7), 869–879.

Tomusiak, A., Strus, M., Heczko, P. B., Adamski, P., Stefański, G., Mikołajczyk-Cichońska, A., & Suda-Szczurek, M. (2015). Efficacy and safety of a vaginal medicinal product containing three strains of probiotic bacteria: A multicenter, randomized, double-blind, and placebo-controlled trial. *Drug Design, Development and Therapy*, *9*, 5345–5354

Torres, N. I., Noll, K. S., Xu, S., Li, J., Huang, Q., Sinko, P. J., … Chikindas, M. L. (2013). Safety, formulation and in vitro antiviral activity of the antimicrobial peptide subtilosin against herpes simplex virus type 1. *Probiotics and Antimicrobial Proteins*, *5*(1), 26–35.

Torriani, S., Van Reenen, C. A., Klein, G., Reuter, G., Dellaglio, F., & Dicks, L. M. T. (1996). *Lactobacillus curvatus* subsp. *curvatus* subsp. nov. and *Lactobacillus curvatus* subsp. *melibiosus* subsp. nov. and *Lactobacillus sake* subsp. *sake* subsp. nov. and *Lactobacillus sake* subsp. carnosus subsp. nov., new subspecies of *Lactobacillus curvatus* Abo-Eln. *International Journal of Systematic Bacteriology*, *46*(4), 1158–1163.

Tuo, Y., Yu, H., Ai, L., Wu, Z., Guo, B., & Chen, W. (2013). Aggregation and adhesion properties of 22 *Lactobacillus* strains. *Journal of Dairy Science*, *96*(7), 4252–4257.

Tyssen, D., Wang, Y., Hayward, J. A., Agius, P. A., Delong, K., Aldunate, M., … Tachedjian, G. (2018). Anti-HIV-1 activity of lactic acid in human cervicovaginal fluid. *American Society for Microbiology*, *3*(4), 1–18.

UNAIDS. (2018). *Report on the global AIDS epidemic 2018.*

Valeriano, V. D., Parungao-Balolong, M. M., & Kang, D. K. (2014). In vitro evaluation of the mucin-adhesion ability and probiotic potential of *Lactobacillus mucosae* LM1. *Journal of Applied Microbiology*, *117*(2), 485–497.

Valore, E. V., Park, C. H., Igreti, S. L., & Ganz, T. (2002). Antimicrobial components of vaginal fluid. *American Journal of Obstetrics and Gynecology*, *187*(3), 561–568.

Van De Wijgert, J. H. H. M., Borgdorff, H., Verhelst, R., Crucitti, T., Francis, S., Verstraelen, H., & Jespers, V. (2014). The vaginal microbiota: What have we learned after a decade of molecular characterisation? *PLoS one*, *9*(8), e105998.

Van de Wijgert, J. H. H. M., & Verwijs, M. C. (2019). Lactobacilli-containing vaginal probiotics to cure or prevent bacterial or fungal vaginal dysbiosis: a systematic review and recommendations for future trial designs. *BJOG: An International Journal of Obstetrics & Gynaecology*, 127(2), 1–13.

Van Houdt, R., Ma, B., Bruisten, S. M., Speksnijder, A. G. C. L., Ravel, J., & De Vries, H. J. C. (2018). *Lactobacillus iners*-dominated vaginal microbiota is associated with increased susceptibility to *Chlamydia trachomatis* infection in Dutch women: A case-control study. *Sexually Transmitted Infections*, *94*(2), 117–123.

Verdenelli, M. C., Cecchini, C., Coman, M. M., Silvi, S., Orpianesi, C., Coata, G., … Di Renzo, G. C. (2016). Impact of probiotic SYNBIO® administered by vaginal suppositories in promoting vaginal health of apparently healthy women. *Current Microbiology*, *73*(4), 483–490.

Verhelst, R., Verstraelen, H., Claeys, G., Verschraegen, G., Delanghe, J., Van Simaey, L., … Vaneechoutte, M. (2004). Cloning of 16S rRNA genes amplified from normal and disturbed vaginal microflora suggests a strong association between *Atopobium vaginae*, *Gardnerella vaginalis* and bacterial vaginosis. *BMC Microbiology*, *4*(16).

Verstraelen, H, Verhelst, R., Claeys, G., De Backer, E., Temmerman, M., & Vaneechoutte, M. (2009). Longitudinal analysis of the vaginal microbiota in pregnancy suggests that *L. crispatus* promotes the stability of the normal vaginal microbiota and that *L. gasseri* and/or *L. iners* are more conducive to the occurrence of abnormal vaginal microbiota. *BMC Microbiol*, *9*(116).

Vitali, B., Abruzzo, A., & Mastromarino, P. (2017). Management of disease and disorders by prebiotics and probiotic therapy: Probiotics in bacterial vaginosis. *The Microbiota in Gastrointestinal Pathophysiology* (399–407).

Vivier, E., Raulet, D. H., Moretta, A., Caligiuri, M. A., Zitvogel, L., Lanier, L. L., … Ugolini, S. (2011). Innate or adaptive immunity? The example of natural killer cells. *Science*, *331*(6013), 44–49.

Wachsman, M. B., Castilla, V., De Ruiz Holgado, A. P., De Torres, R. A., Sesma, F., & Coto, C. E. (2003). Enterocin CRL35 inhibits late stages of HSV-1 and HSV-2 replication in vitro. *Antiviral Research*, *58*(1), 17–24.

Wagner, R. D., Johnson, S. J., & Tucker, D. R. (2012). Protection of vaginal epithelial cells with probiotic lactobacilli and the effect of estrogen against infection by *Candida albicans*; *Open Journal of Medical Microbiology*, *02*(03), 54–64.

Wang, G., Xia, Y., Cui, J., Gu, Z., Song, Y., Chen, Y. Q., … Chen, W. (2014). The roles of moonlighting proteins in bacteria. *Current Issues in Molecular Biology*, *16*(1), 15–22.

Wang, G., Zhang, M., Zhao, J., Xia, Y., Lai, P. F. H., & Ai, L. (2018). A surface protein from *Lactobacillus plantarum* increases the adhesion of *Lactobacillus* strains to human epithelial cells. *Frontiers in Microbiology*, *9*(NOV), 1–9.

Wang, J., Wu, R., Zhang, W., Sun, Z., Zhao, W., & Zhang, H. (2013). Proteomic comparison of the probiotic bacterium *Lactobacillus casei* cultivated in milk and soy milk. *Journal of Dairy Science*, *96*(9), 5603–5624.

Waśko, A., Polak-Berecka, M., Paduch, R., & Jóźwiak, K. (2014). The effect of moonlighting proteins on the adhesion and aggregation ability of *Lactobacillus helveticus*. *Anaerobe*, *30*, 161–168.

Weiss, R. A. (1993). Cellular receptors and viral glycoproteins involved in retrovirus entry. *The Retroviridae*, 1–108.

Weissenhorn, W., Dessen, A., SC, H., JJ, S., & DC, W. (1997). Atomic-structure of the ectodomain from HIV-1 Gp41. *Nature*, *387*(6631), 426–430.

Weng, S.-L., Chiu, C.-M., Lin, F.-M., Huang, W.-C., Liang, C., Yang, T., … Huang, H.-D. (2014). Bacterial communities in semen from men of infertile couples: metagenomic sequencing reveals relationships of seminal microbiota to semen quality. *PLoS one*, *9*(10), e110152.

Wertz, J., Isaacs-Cosgrove, N., Holzman, C., & Marsh, T. L. (2008). Temporal shifts in microbial communities in nonpregnant African-American women with and without bacterial vaginosis. *Interdisciplinary Perspectives on Infectious Diseases*, *2008(181253)*, 1–9.

WHO. (2002). *FAO/WHO. Guidelines for the evaluation of probiotics in food. Food and Health Agricultural Organization of the United Nations and World Health Organization. Working Group Report.*

Wiesenfeld, H. C., Hillier, S. L., Krohn, M. A., Landers, D. V., & Sweet, R. L. (2003). Bacterial vaginosis is a strong predictor of *Neisseria gonorrhoeae* and *Chlamydia trachomatis* infection. *Clinical Infectious Diseases*, *36*(5), 663–668.

Wiesner, J., & Vilcinskas, A. (2010). Antimicrobial peptides: The ancient arm of the human immune system. *Virulence*, *1*(5), 440–464.

Williams, B., Landay, A., & Presti, R. M. (2016). Microbiome alterations in HIV infection a review, *Cellular microbiology, 18*(5), 645–651.

Wira, C R, Fahey, J. V, Sentman, C. L., Pioli, P. A., & Shen, L. (2005). Innate and adaptive immunity in female genital tract: cellular responses and interactions. *Immunological Reviews*, *206*(0105-2896 (Print)), 306–335.

Wira, Charles R., Fahey, J. V., Ghosh, M., Patel, M. V., Hickey, D. K., & Ochiel, D. O. (2010). Sex hormone regulation of innate immunity in the female reproductive tract: The role of epithelial cells in balancing reproductive potential with protection against sexually transmitted pathogens. *American Journal of Reproductive Immunology*, *63*(6), 544–565.

Witkin, S. S. (2015). The vaginal microbiome, vaginal anti-microbial defence mechanisms and the clinical challenge of reducing infection-related preterm birth. *BJOG: An International Journal of Obstetrics and Gynaecology*, *122*(2), 213–218.

Witkin, Steven S., Linhares, I. M., & Giraldo, P. (2007). Bacterial flora of the female genital tract: function and immune regulation. *Best Practice and Research: Clinical Obstetrics and Gynaecology*, *21*(3), 347–354.

Witkin, Steven S., Mendes-Soares, M., L. I., Jayaram Aswathi, J, L. W., & Forney Larry J. (2013). Influence of vaginal bacteria and D- and L-lactic acid isomers on vaginal extracellular matrix metalloproteinase inducer: implications for protection against upper genital tract infections. *American Society for Microbiology*, *4*(4), 1–7.

Wu, Z., Chen, Z., & Phillips, D. M. (2003). Human genital epithelial cells capture cell-free human immunodeficiency virus type 1 and transmit the virus to CD4+ cells: implications for mechanisms of sexual transmission. *The Journal of Infectious Diseases*, *188*(10), 1473–1482.

Wyatt, R., & Sodroski, J. (1998). The HIV-1 envelope glycoproteins: Fusogens, antigens, and immunogens. *Science*, *280*(5371), 1884–1888.

Yadav, A. K., Tyagi, A., Kumar, A., Panwar, S., Grover, S., Saklani, A. C., … Batish, V. K. (2017). Adhesion of lactobacilli and their anti-infectivity potential. *Critical Reviews in Food Science and Nutrition*, *57*(10), 2042–2056.

Yamamoto, T., Zhou, X., Williams, C. J., Hochwalt, A., & Forney, L. J. (2009). Bacterial populations in the vaginas of healthy adolescent women. *Journal of Pediatric and Adolescent Gynecology*, *22*(1), 11–18.

Yazdi, A. S., & Goreschi, K. (2016). The Interleukin-1 Family. *Regulation of Cytokine Gene Expression in Immunity and Diseases* (pp. 21–29).

Yeoman, C. J., Thomas, S. M., Miller, M. E. B., Ulanov, A. V., Torralba, M., Lucas, S., … White, B. A. (2013). A multi-omic systems-based approach reveals metabolic markers of bacterial vaginosis and insight into the disease. *PLoS one*, *8*(2), e56111.

Yeoman, C. J., Yildirim, S., Thomas, S. M., Durkin, A. S., Torralba, M., Sutton, G., … Wilson, B. A. (2010). Comparative genomics of *Gardnerella vaginalis* strains reveals substantial differences in metabolic and virulence potential. *PLoS one*, *5*(8), e12411.

Zalán, Z., Hudáček, J., Štětina, J., Chumchalová, J., & Halász, A. (2010). Production of organic acids by *Lactobacillus* strains in three different media. *European Food Research and Technology*, *230*(3), 395–404.

Zariffard, M. R., Novak, R. M., Lurain, N., Sha, B. E., Graham, P., & Spear, G. T. (2005). Induction of tumor necrosis factor–α secretion and toll-like receptor 2 and 4 mRNA expression by genital mucosal fluids from women with bacterial vaginosis. *The Journal of Infectious Diseases*, *191*(11), 1913–1921.

Zevin, A. S., Xie, I. Y., Birse, K., Arnold, K., Romas, L., Westmacott, G., … Burgener, A. D. (2016). Microbiome composition and function drives wound-healing impairment in the female genital tract. *PLoS Pathogens*, *12*(9), 1–20.

Zhai, Z., Douillard, F. P., An, H., Wang, G., Guo, X., Luo, Y., & Hao, Y. (2014). Proteomic characterisation of the acid tolerance response in *Lactobacillus delbrueckii* subsp. *bulgaricus* CAUH1 and functional identification of a novel acid stress-related transcriptional regulator Ldb0677. *Environmental Microbiology*, *16*(6), 1524–1537.

Zhang, W., Wang, H., Liu, J., Zhao, Y., Gao, K., & Zhang, J. (2013). Adhesive ability means inhibition activities for *Lactobacillus* against pathogens and S-layer protein plays an important role in adhesion. *Anaerobe*, *22*, 97–103.

Zhang, Y., Liu, Y., Ma, Q., Song, Y., Zhang, Q., Wang, X., & Chen, F. (2014). Identification of *Lactobacillus* from the saliva of adult patients with caries using matrix-assisted laser desorption/ionization time-of-flight mass spectrometry. *PLoS one*, *9*(8), 3–9.

Zhou, X, Brown, C. J., Abdo, Z., Davis, C. C., Hansmann, M. A., Joyce, P., … Forney, L. J. (2007). Differences in the composition of vaginal microbial communities found in healthy Caucasian and black women. *International Society for Microbial Ecology*, *1*(121-133).

Zhou, Xia, Bent, S. J., Schneider, M. G., Davis, C. C., Islam, M. R., & Forney, L. J. (2004). Characterisation of vaginal microbial communities in adult healthy women using cultivation-independent methods. *Microbiology*, *150*(8), 2565–2573.

Zoetendal, E. G., von Wright, A., Vilpponen-Salmela, T., Ben-Amor, K., Akkermans, A. D. L., & de Vos, W. M. (2002). Mucosa-associated bacteria in the human gastrointestinal tract are uniformly distributed along the colon and differ from the community recovered from feces. *Applied and Environmental Microbiology*, *68*(7), 3401–3407.

Appendix I : Preparation of reagents

MRS broth

Five hundred milliliters of distilled water were warmed for 5 minutes in a microwave. Fifty grams of MRS powder (Sigma Aldrich, USA), 50mg of Cystein (Sigma Aldrich, USA) and 1ml of Tween 80 (Sigma-Aldrich, USA) was added to the warmed water and stirred until dissolved well. The mixture was topped up to a 1L with distilled water and mixed well. The media was poured into sterile 500ml Schott bottles, labeled and autoclaved at 121°C for 15 minutes. The broth was allowed to cool and then stored in the fridge at 4°C.

MRS-agar

MRS broth was prepared as described above, but before autoclaving, 2.4g of Bacto-agar (Sigma-Aldrich, USA) was added to 200ml of MRS in a sterile 500ml Schott bottle. The bottles were labeled and autoclaved at 121°C for 15 minutes before being allowed to cool. The media was stored in the fridge at 4°C.

Brain Heart Infusion (BHI) broth preparation

Five hundred mililitres of distilled water were warmed in the microwave. Thirty-seven grams of BHI powder (Sigma-Aldrich, USA), 10g of yeast extract (Sigma-Aldrich, USA) and 1g of soluble starch (Sigma-Aldrich, USA) were added to the warm distilled water and gently swirled until well dissolved before being autoclaved at 121°C for 15 minutes. After autoclaving, the media was allowed to cool before aseptically aliquoting into sterile 20ml culture and stored at 4°C.

Shaedler blood agar preparation

Five hundred milliliters of distilled water were warmed in the microwave before dissolving 26.5g of Shaedler's broth powder (Sigma-Aldrich, USA) and 12g of Bacto agar (Sigma-Aldrich, USA). The broth mixture was autoclaved at 121°C for 15 minutes. After autoclaving, the media was allowed to cool before aseptically adding 50 ml of defibrinated horse blood (final concentration 5%).

Columbia blood culture medium

Five hundred milliliters of distilled water were warmed in the microwave before dissolving 19.5g of Columbia broth powder (Sigma-Aldrich, USA) and 12g of Bacto agar (Sigma-Aldrich, USA). The broth mixture was autoclaved at 121°C for 15 minutes. After autoclaving, the media was allowed to cool before aseptically adding 50 ml of defibrinated horse blood (final concentration 5%).

Gram-stain protocol

To prepare smears on microscope slides for Gram staining, single drops of saline were placed on each slide. Sterile loops were used to pick single colonies from culture plates and resuspended in the saline before preparing smears on the slides. The slides were heat-fixed, covered with crystal violet solution for one minute, after which the solution was rinsed off with tap water. The same process was repeated with iodine solution. The slides were then flooded with decolorizer for 5 seconds, rinsed with water, flooded with safranin for 30 seconds and rinsed in tap water. The slides were dried gently with paper towel before being microscopically examined under a 1000x objective.

Appendix II: Gram stained images of lactobacilli strains

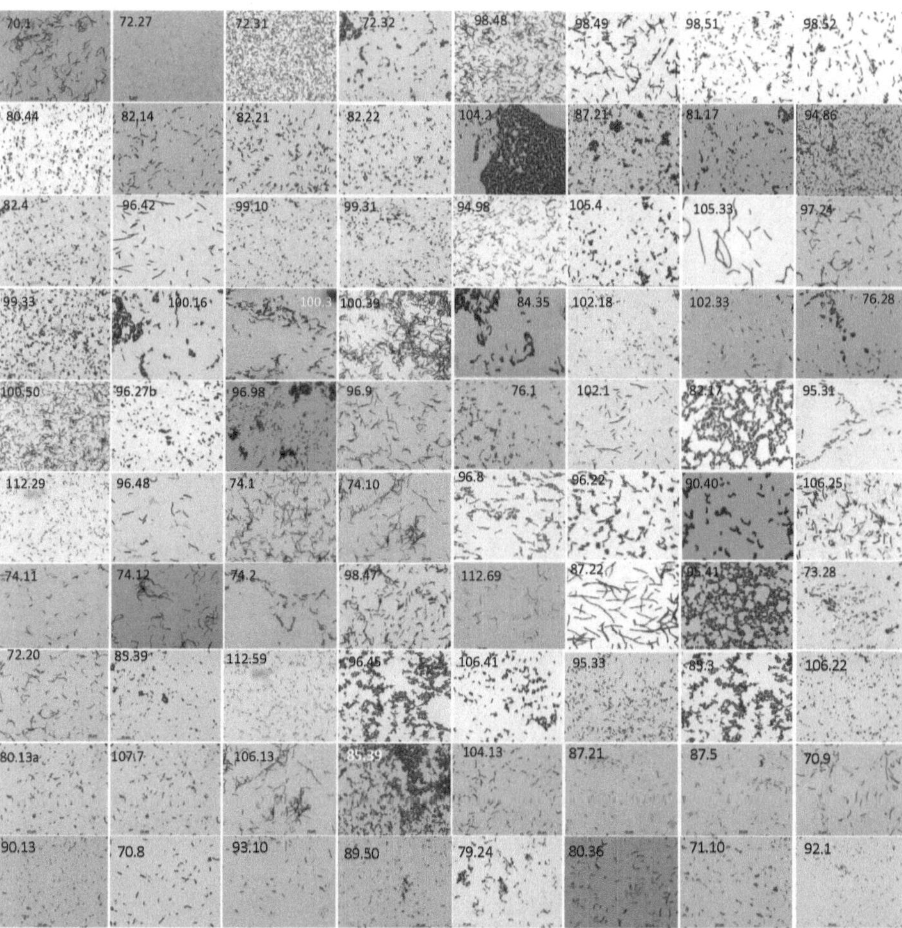

Appendix II shows Gram stained images of lactobacilli isolates. The numbers on the images represent the lactobacilli strain numbers. The species names can be found in Figure 3.1 in Chapter 3.

Appendix III: Gram stained images showing adhesion of lactobacilli strains to VK2 cells

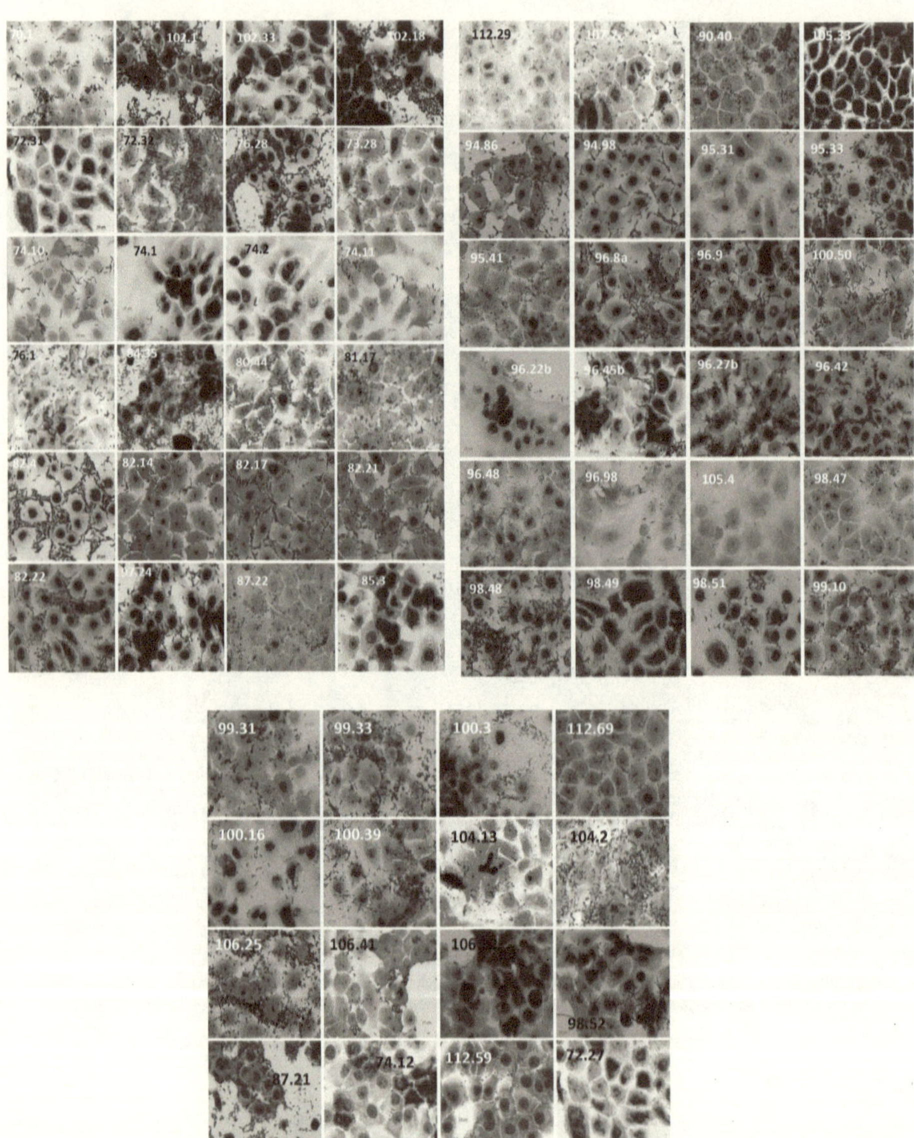

Appendix IV : Table S1. List of differentially abundant proteins between lactobacilli inducing low versus high inflammation

Protein IDs	logFC	AveExpr	t	P.Value	adj.P.Val	B
F4AF14	-4.9486995	0.47434975	-6.0435617	2.37E-07	0.00120377	6.68652493
C4VLF8	-4.7532612	1.63686742	-5.521565	1.44E-06	0.00366283	5.0672866
F4AGA9	-4.1806702	0.39932164	-5.1953486	4.40E-06	0.00745552	4.06477744
F4AGJ4	-4.7511507	2.41245272	-5.098478	6.12E-06	0.00776909	3.76928757
G2SMT3	-4.0809295	0.04046474	-4.9682364	9.50E-06	0.00813052	3.37397328
C4VL06	-4.5885036	1.02288611	-4.9238088	1.10E-05	0.00813052	3.23969213
D6S2W7	-4.5187913	1.27110534	-4.9191528	1.12E-05	0.00813052	3.22563735
A0A2I1XR25	-4.7199898	3.21218167	-4.8524476	1.40E-05	0.00889789	3.02465983
C4VKY3	-4.226816	0.45672712	-4.7515224	1.96E-05	0.00954192	2.72201547
F4ACD9	-3.7125427	3.71076034	-4.7401822	2.04E-05	0.00954192	2.68812356
C4VLP0	-4.1991855	2.86539957	-4.6983633	2.34E-05	0.00954192	2.56334951
C4VK70	-3.8356906	0.24610087	-4.6585326	2.67E-05	0.00954192	2.44481942
C4VNZ5	-4.1706104	0.72097421	-4.6418148	2.82E-05	0.00954192	2.39516311
C4VN38	-4.4606941	2.20201778	-4.6232309	3.00E-05	0.00954192	2.34003015
F4AG33	-4.3567138	1.75947204	-4.6064537	3.17E-05	0.00954192	2.29031767
C4VN26	-4.3418702	2.08750037	-4.5885237	3.37E-05	0.00954192	2.23725364
F4ACU4	-4.1733656	1.62431561	-4.5759436	3.51E-05	0.00954192	2.20006307
C4VN24	-4.3230114	1.77780189	-4.5578815	3.73E-05	0.00954192	2.14672483
F4AE87	-4.3215864	1.13906859	-4.5562406	3.75E-05	0.00954192	2.14188248
F4AEY3	-4.1904264	1.04774761	-4.5430439	3.91E-05	0.00954192	2.10296107
C4VLF1	-4.967675	2.76648488	-4.5404952	3.94E-05	0.00954192	2.09544842
F4AFC8	-4.0023462	2.85590525	-4.514229	4.30E-05	0.00979626	2.01810827
F4AEC2	-5.1471891	1.82143293	-4.4992017	4.52E-05	0.00979626	1.97392962
C4VKJ3	-4.807701	1.54644514	-4.481167	4.79E-05	0.00979626	1.92097674
C4VN07	-4.3753933	3.31781071	-4.4672043	5.02E-05	0.00979626	1.88003079
C4VKD6	-3.9080083	0.61955874	-4.4576039	5.18E-05	0.00979626	1.85190361
D6S5W5	-4.49721	3.02255465	-4.4557358	5.21E-05	0.00979626	1.84643277
D6S470	-4.6867275	3.30420143	-4.3917734	6.41E-05	0.01163492	1.65961676
D6S2V4	-4.3732172	1.28535104	-4.3604355	7.10E-05	0.01243664	1.56844857
C4VPM0	-3.9054579	3.09777795	-4.3445606	7.47E-05	0.01265666	1.52235825
C4VL99	-3.3804982	-0.0351763	-4.3176148	8.16E-05	0.01336391	1.44427066
F4AGS3	-4.3774169	1.30332793	-4.2993743	8.65E-05	0.01373169	1.3915162
F4AC26	-3.6940758	0.18475317	-4.2694991	9.52E-05	0.01464255	1.30529957
F4AGH9	-4.1567381	2.3769539	-4.2553325	9.97E-05	0.01464255	1.26449859
D6S4K6	-5.1078271	3.38653275	-4.2449749	1.03E-04	0.01464255	1.2347017
C4VP45	-4.2756429	1.41764129	-4.2428342	1.04E-04	0.01464255	1.22854702
Q1WS45	4.46229105	0.66484857	4.2334759	1.07E-04	0.01468131	1.20165536
D6S2H4	-4.4379045	1.59045139	-4.2106959	1.15E-04	0.01501124	1.13629527

F4AEX4	-3.7785019	5.20192537	-4.2101222	1.15E-04	0.01501124	1.13465096
F4AEV6	-4.0694625	2.33702765	-4.1667766	1.32E-04	0.01656871	1.01068818
C4VNH0	-4.4412603	1.96787672	-4.1635892	1.34E-04	0.01656871	1.00159359
C4VMP7	-4.2507379	2.53362117	-4.1513906	1.39E-04	0.0167672	0.96681366
F4ACS4	-4.0120819	0.70170316	-4.1327682	1.48E-04	0.0167672	0.91380123
A0A2I1XN99	-4.0355035	0.72806803	-4.1310296	1.48E-04	0.0167672	0.90885696
F4AGP0	-4.8043086	1.96259508	-4.1270476	1.50E-04	0.0167672	0.89753636
D6S3E4	-4.0415618	1.97712511	-4.118675	1.54E-04	0.0167672	0.87374885
F4AFE6	-3.8267617	0.58657848	-4.1169397	1.55E-04	0.0167672	0.86882092
F4AG36	-3.802736	1.7420398	-4.0936943	1.67E-04	0.01736248	0.80289734
D6S5Q9	-4.9455561	2.11729374	-4.0928091	1.67E-04	0.01736248	0.80039023
D6S474	-5.0147596	2.18671748	-4.0792963	1.75E-04	0.01775926	0.7621454
C4VNJ6	-4.0297753	3.82740882	-4.0673586	1.82E-04	0.01808113	0.72840387
C4VLP6	-3.6801058	1.32830761	-4.0609083	1.85E-04	0.01809866	0.71019038
C4VMK6	-3.454747	5.0843345	-4.0475031	1.93E-04	0.01820333	0.67237893
C4VNT0	-3.8711963	1.20465745	-4.04713	1.93E-04	0.01820333	0.67132745
F9ULM5	-3.7556157	2.51282624	-4.0361537	2.00E-04	0.01850191	0.64040908
Q1WSB4	4.07447045	0.77202458	4.02805029	2.05E-04	0.01864149	0.61760708
F4AFI6	-4.1031718	1.10388725	-4.0142845	2.15E-04	0.01887479	0.5789184
A0A226U5K4	-3.6784531	0.15556287	-4.0129498	2.15E-04	0.01887479	0.57517033
C4VM62	-3.9282335	1.2723958	-4.0069256	2.20E-04	0.01890969	0.55826056
A0A2I1XN25	-4.3190959	1.62595648	-3.9970257	2.27E-04	0.01908156	0.5304965
C4VNP0	-3.8581478	2.88098819	-3.9934326	2.29E-04	0.01908156	0.52042733
C4VK73	-3.8593577	1.52425788	-3.9826027	2.37E-04	0.01942266	0.49010262
F4AG30	-3.8229941	1.22196351	-3.9679521	2.48E-04	0.0200123	0.44913936
F4AEZ3	-3.7975148	3.35851209	-3.9591458	2.55E-04	0.02025011	0.42454989
C4VLA0	-3.9020506	3.76770136	-3.9524233	2.61E-04	0.02036219	0.40579572
C4VLK4	-3.6845428	2.27210243	-3.9348334	2.75E-04	0.02118627	0.35679367
F4AFR9	-3.9139748	3.8263659	-3.9217043	2.87E-04	0.02165154	0.32028444
D6S478	-4.0661819	4.83674133	-3.9130395	2.95E-04	0.02165154	0.29622069
C4VN98	-4.0064615	2.07339888	-3.912739	2.95E-04	0.02165154	0.29538669
F4AD91	-3.9164055	1.35116383	-3.9089826	2.98E-04	0.02165154	0.28496244
C4VL86	-3.5897135	2.19925986	-3.8865968	3.20E-04	0.02284425	0.22293868
C4VME3	-4.3620586	1.72571192	-3.8826655	3.24E-04	0.02284425	0.21206381
F4AD51	-3.9067883	3.06184149	-3.8758051	3.31E-04	0.02301603	0.19309884
F4AGJ2	-3.7748109	3.71782717	-3.8535791	3.54E-04	0.02422832	0.13176647
C4VN18	-3.5650711	0.15671643	-3.8505052	3.58E-04	0.02422832	0.12329716
C4VMS3	-4.3016574	3.04150603	-3.8311072	3.80E-04	0.02538635	0.06992777
C4VLD3	-3.6741245	0.5081354	-3.8048585	4.12E-04	0.02672971	-0.0020813
C4VLS3	-2.7435048	4.50967367	-3.8021657	4.15E-04	0.02672971	-0.009455
F4AFY7	-3.0853566	-0.4573217	-3.8006436	4.17E-04	0.02672971	-0.0136218

F4AF81	-4.1797328	3.00551331	-3.7964466	4.23E-04	0.02672971	-0.0251069
D6S4W9	-2.8921775	-0.5539112	-3.7913927	4.29E-04	0.02672971	-0.0389287
C4VLA7	-3.6049029	4.8166345	-3.7852773	4.37E-04	0.02672971	-0.0556413
F4AFX6	-3.5891107	1.90784831	-3.7823596	4.41E-04	0.02672971	-0.0636103
C4VL05	-4.1411183	2.49617681	-3.7818405	4.42E-04	0.02672971	-0.0650276
F4AD84	-3.3400434	0.27984039	-3.7737004	4.53E-04	0.02708329	-0.0872429
C4VMN8	-2.5724633	4.62354144	-3.7680423	4.61E-04	0.02722498	-0.1026705
F4ADM3	-3.5382669	0.66122619	-3.7644106	4.66E-04	0.02722498	-0.1125667
D6S5P5	-3.8276827	0.91863219	-3.7467453	4.92E-04	0.02841083	-0.1606359
D6S669	-3.5408075	0.44187003	-3.7379062	5.06E-04	0.02868366	-0.1846452
F4AEG3	-3.2085105	0.19046123	-3.7362625	5.08E-04	0.02868366	-0.1891068
G2SLR2	3.27020682	0.01346491	3.7251272	5.26E-04	0.02934902	-0.2193061
C4VM39	-3.8541836	1.25281214	-3.7199333	5.34E-04	0.02949336	-0.2333764
G2SMN8	3.81397316	1.58416006	3.70332728	5.62E-04	0.0306894	-0.2782953
C4VPB9	-3.8626616	2.73401101	-3.6947654	5.77E-04	0.03116368	-0.3014148
C4VMP4	-3.9242736	1.65789155	-3.6781214	6.07E-04	0.03167834	-0.3462799
A0A2M9WNZ3	-3.5638138	0.49590452	-3.6780385	6.07E-04	0.03167834	-0.346503
C4VL34	-3.8428675	3.36358578	-3.6767299	6.09E-04	0.03167834	-0.3500258
F4AC50	-3.6388815	2.0737631	-3.6756398	6.11E-04	0.03167834	-0.35296
F4ADM4	-3.672699	3.21245295	-3.6591681	6.42E-04	0.03264644	-0.3972418
C4VMS4	-3.6891611	1.15654442	-3.6569853	6.47E-04	0.03264644	-0.4031022
D6S4L6	-3.5249699	3.02089198	-3.6557418	6.49E-04	0.03264644	-0.4064401
C4VKC6	-3.6404301	3.19033294	-3.6410592	6.79E-04	0.03379295	-0.4458055
F4ADB5	-3.5066224	0.44967854	-3.632877	6.95E-04	0.03407493	-0.4677066
F4AEJ2	-3.1078458	-0.1738458	-3.63187	6.98E-04	0.03407493	-0.4704003
C4VP92	-4.0694596	0.89495496	-3.6233858	7.16E-04	0.03451844	-0.4930792
C4VP36	-3.670082	0.86399604	-3.6187829	7.26E-04	0.03451844	-0.5053713
F4AD95	-3.7225281	2.83409506	-3.617506	7.28E-04	0.03451844	-0.5087797
C4VMS2	-3.5641674	1.69668766	-3.6082275	7.49E-04	0.03451844	-0.5335285
C4VNZ2	-3.8128801	2.9530463	-3.5989598	7.70E-04	0.03451844	-0.5582146
D6S4W0	-3.8171162	1.31746507	-3.597515	7.74E-04	0.03451844	-0.5620602
D6S423	-4.4070578	1.16161321	-3.5968441	7.75E-04	0.03451844	-0.5638453
C4VPL2	-3.9048826	1.7161035	-3.5962467	7.77E-04	0.03451844	-0.5654351
F9UTQ7	-4.04464	2.03522032	-3.5950767	7.79E-04	0.03451844	-0.5685479
F4AF66	-3.3277719	1.44180592	-3.5946722	7.80E-04	0.03451844	-0.5696239
F4AGB8	-3.4509387	2.97953872	-3.5941545	7.81E-04	0.03451844	-0.5710011
C4VLU3	-3.9228714	1.41209148	-3.589446	7.93E-04	0.03459888	-0.583521
C4VLT6	-3.7184091	1.87400837	-3.586842	7.99E-04	0.03459888	-0.5904414
Q88X05	-3.8079817	2.14538189	-3.5844334	8.05E-04	0.03459888	-0.5968401
C4VNA1	-3.2424279	-0.0504383	-3.5819784	8.10E-04	0.03459888	-0.6033596
C4VMA4	-4.0287068	1.20791144	-3.5661653	8.50E-04	0.03586065	-0.6452956

A0A2I1XNH1	-3.7201542	0.93597464	-3.5612743	8.62E-04	0.03586065	-0.6582463
C4VPJ7	-4.3044353	1.11225126	-3.5580712	8.71E-04	0.03586065	-0.6667223
C4VPC1	-4.0938989	1.25729278	-3.5562572	8.75E-04	0.03586065	-0.6715208
C4VLN5	-3.8318401	2.0319102	-3.5551853	8.78E-04	0.03586065	-0.6743556
F4AGQ5	-3.5432865	2.65610916	-3.5535613	8.82E-04	0.03586065	-0.6786494
F4AEY7	-3.1095035	-0.1247483	-3.5478132	8.98E-04	0.0361917	-0.6938392
C4VPL5	-4.0620404	2.48289913	-3.5326109	9.39E-04	0.03707818	-0.7339483
D6S5V6	-3.3930337	4.99429094	-3.5323539	9.40E-04	0.03707818	-0.7346254
C4VKC7	-3.3479516	0.04364436	-3.5318004	9.42E-04	0.03707818	-0.7360838
F4ACJ4	-3.6000375	1.29205451	-3.5248049	9.61E-04	0.0373706	-0.7545065
Q1WUY7	3.69583302	0.24812728	3.52399133	9.64E-04	0.0373706	-0.7566477
C4VMF1	-3.7189874	2.86109804	-3.520194	9.75E-04	0.03750867	-0.7666382
C4VNX7	-3.5398456	3.93256945	-3.5128369	9.96E-04	0.03804948	-0.7859777
F4AEX2	-2.4341555	6.44073458	-3.5063477	1.02E-03	0.03849025	-0.8030171
K1MDU1	-3.0180321	-0.1583333	-3.5039287	1.02E-03	0.03849025	-0.8093645
F9UPK7	-4.3792917	3.54887181	-3.4946042	1.05E-03	0.0389826	-0.833809
C4VNG1	-4.0373074	1.57527055	-3.4939363	1.05E-03	0.0389826	-0.8355584
A0A3E7	3.3367348	1.23991241	3.4922264	1.06E-03	0.0389826	-0.8400366
D6S4C4	-3.8640961	1.78011826	-3.480254	1.10E-03	0.03970538	-0.8713578
F4AGS1	-3.0808778	-0.4595611	-3.4785227	1.10E-03	0.03970538	-0.8758821
C4VN39	-3.0667118	-0.1173611	-3.4758074	1.11E-03	0.03970538	-0.8829755
Q1WS90	3.61847215	1.16705845	3.47448504	1.12E-03	0.03970538	-0.8864287
F4AFW8	-3.6643291	2.31543698	-3.473986	1.12E-03	0.03970538	-0.8877318
F4ADU0	-2.8638421	4.31155285	-3.4632951	1.15E-03	0.04069413	-0.9156215
C4VNA5	-3.3101075	0.2946201	-3.4586188	1.17E-03	0.04087422	-0.9278057
F4ADH7	-3.3288286	0.97518532	-3.457121	1.17E-03	0.04087422	-0.9317062
D6S486	-2.5653333	5.92109086	-3.4516181	1.19E-03	0.04099081	-0.9460285
F4AEN3	-2.8185431	-0.5907285	-3.4502003	1.20E-03	0.04099081	-0.9497168
F4AFE2	-3.2199598	3.01907738	-3.4460463	1.21E-03	0.04099081	-0.9605172
C4VMR8	-2.6323077	-0.6838462	-3.4459672	1.21E-03	0.04099081	-0.960723
D6S3Z5	-3.0388193	5.93049093	-3.4416305	1.23E-03	0.04099081	-0.9719905
F4AET2	-4.1835248	3.34706112	-3.4405426	1.23E-03	0.04099081	-0.974816
F4AEG2	-2.6574613	-0.6712694	-3.4402493	1.23E-03	0.04099081	-0.9755775
P71478	-4.1313996	2.87664132	-3.4261283	1.29E-03	0.0422387	-1.0122029
C4VPJ0	-3.5065706	0.45136424	-3.4256225	1.29E-03	0.0422387	-1.0135133
F4AGW4	-3.4866982	2.52496721	-3.4224328	1.30E-03	0.04236262	-1.0217738
F4ADM5	-3.4243718	3.41528808	-3.4035443	1.37E-03	0.0444415	-1.0706002
K1N0L4	-3.3295932	0.34701897	-3.4017318	1.38E-03	0.0444415	-1.0752774
C4VL27	-3.199928	0.25549717	-3.3892084	1.43E-03	0.04580842	-1.107555
F4AEC3	-3.9864067	2.18641448	-3.3793375	1.48E-03	0.04673093	-1.1329478
C4VNJ9	-3.1719354	3.91387301	-3.3780913	1.48E-03	0.04673093	-1.1361505

A0A2I1XN33	-2.9187949	0.05241475	-3.3627906	1.55E-03	0.0485588	-1.1754179
C4VKL1	-3.244092	0.3046539	-3.3532333	1.59E-03	0.04962062	-1.1998932
C4VMF0	-3.330098	5.07728179	-3.3489192	1.61E-03	0.04993986	-1.2109279

www.ingramcontent.com/pod-product-compliance
Lightning Source LLC
LaVergne TN
LVHW091311150826

845673LV00006B/1612
9783384245045